# The Hundred-Year Diet

# The Hundred-Year Diet

✦

## Guidelines and Recipes for a Long and Vigorous Life


*Blair Beebe, MD*

*Former Associate Executive Director,*
*The Permanente Medical Group, Kaiser Permanente*

*Sue Beebe, MA*

*French-Trained Culinary Expert*



iUniverse, Inc.

New York Bloomington

# The Hundred-Year DIET
## Guidelines and Recipes for a Long and Vigorous Life



iUniverse books may be ordered through booksellers or by contacting:

iUniverse
1663 Liberty Drive
Bloomington, IN 47403
www.iuniverse.com
1-800-Authors (1-800-288-4677)

ISBN: 978-0-595-48678-6 (pbk)
ISBN: 978-0-595-48985-5 (cloth)
ISBN: 978-0-595-60774-7 (ebk)

Printed in the United States of America

iUniverse rev. date: 11/12/08

*Dedicated to our children*

*Blair*
*Helen*
*John*
*Sarah*

*Don't look back! Something might be gaining on you.*

—Satchel Paige

# *Contents*

Recipes

Soup



Seafood



Poultry

Pasta, Rice, and Couscous



Asian Food



Vegetables



Bread

# *Preface*

We Americans are the most hospitalized people in the world; one in every thousand of us will spend today in a hospital bed. In more than half of these cases, we could have prevented that hospitalization with sound health-promoting practices; but we continue with our bad habits because of a confusing and conflicting barrage of advice. Should we restrict fat or restrict carbohydrates in our diet? Is butter better than stick margarine?

A major purpose of this book is to explain the evidence behind advice about weight control and disease prevention, and then to present a sensible plan for action that includes recipes for better nutrition and basic information about exercise. Some popular self-help books promote recommendations that are no more than speculation, which means that the advice may be good—and then again it may not be. On the other hand, the scientific literature contains a huge number of clinical trials with measurable results that document whether or not specific recommendations lead to effective weight control and enhance good health.

In *The One Hundred-Year Diet,* we have tried to present the evidence in an easily readable fashion, so readers may decide for themselves what is most important. For anyone who wishes to read the primary scientific references, we've included citations for every major recommendation. Most of the original articles are accessible online through Medline at the Web site of the National Library of Medicine (www.nlm.nih.gov).

The preventive medicine philosophy that we present in the book comes from many years in practice with my Kaiser Permanente colleagues in California. The founders of the Permanente Medical Group were passionate about prevention of disease and maintenance of good health. Today's Permanente physicians continue to support that preventive philosophy with large numbers of health education programs that we still offer to our patients; and as a result, Kaiser Permanente patients have a lower mortality rate than the general population from serious degenerative diseases. For example, heart disease is no longer the number one cause of death among our patients as it is in the rest of the country.

My wife Sue and I live in a small community next to Stanford University where, earlier in my career, I had been a member of the clinical faculty in the Department of Endocrinology and Metabolism. Sue is a microbiologist with an interest in nutrition on a cellular basis that stems from studying microorganisms. She has taught nursing students at nearby San Jose State University and two local community colleges. As our four children left for college, Sue sent each of them with a notebook of handwritten recipes illustrating examples of healthful nutrition. They all still use them, and two of our children have won prizes for their own recipes published in *Better Homes and Gardens.*

Because of the agreeable climate, we ride bicycles year round and work out four times a week with a Pacific Masters swimming group. For *The Hundred-Year Diet*, we have added practical tips from our own experiences in physical fitness and nutrition to the large volume of published scientific literature.

Blair Beebe, MD
Portola Valley, California
2008

# PART I
## Guidelines for Healthful Living

# *Introduction*

Today's normal average life expectancy from birth should be about one hundred years; so why do we live only to 77.9 years, according to the National Center for Health Statistics? And, why do some elderly Americans spend so many years disabled? The answer is that most of us succumb to preventable degenerative illnesses that cause early disability and death, like heart disease, strokes, and diabetes. Many of us don't realize that we're at risk, because those diseases defy early detection. For example, the first indication of heart disease might be a fatal heart attack. While not always avoidable, most degenerative diseases can be delayed, and sometimes completely prevented, by developing a few basic health-promoting habits.

A report from the United States Bureau of the Census notes that "the number of centenarians is exploding," and forecasts a long-term increase of about twenty-five years in life expectancy from birth in future centuries, "which some experts today believe to be quite conservative" (Kinsella 2005, S299–S303). Other long-term average life-expectancy projections range from age eighty-seven (Wilmoth 2000, 1111–1129) to 120 years (Luria 2005, S317–319). Although they may disagree about life-span predictions, all geriatricians agree that improvements in preventive health habits would result in a substantial increase in longevity and a reduction in the prevalence of old-age disability (Olshansky 1990, 634–640). Pessimistic forecasts for widespread adaptation of better health habits underlie the shorter life-expectancy projections, while the optimistic estimates depend upon significantly more attention to health promotion than exists today.

Many people believe that robust health depends only upon fate and good genes, and that we have little control over our future well-being. A study from Johns Hopkins University showed that older adults who attributed functional decline to "old age" actually suffered from specific conditions that were potentially preventable (Williamson 1996, 1429–1434). While genetic predisposition and bad luck underlie some diseases, we can take steps to reduce our risk of many causes of early disability and death, including almost all of the major degenerative diseases.

*The Hundred-Year Diet* reviews the principles of disease prevention with an emphasis on reducing risk factors that pose the greatest danger to good health. Although it does not pretend to offer a magic formula for fast weight reduction, following the nutritional guidelines consistently will result in a more permanent normalization of weight. Strong evidence supports the conclusion that a poor diet underlies many serious chronic diseases. A healthful diet should be an integral part of a long-term, comprehensive health-promoting program that includes:

- Reaching and maintaining an ideal weight
- Improving blood cholesterol levels
- Controlling blood pressure
- Reducing blood sugar levels if diabetes is present
- Eliminating smoking
- Participating in daily vigorous exercise

Every five years since 1980, the Office of Disease Prevention and Health Promotion of the Department of Health and Human Services has sponsored a blue-ribbon panel of clinical experts to comb the scientific literature on nutrition, exercise, and other forms of health promotion.[1] They determine whether sufficient evidence exists to draw conclusions about specific recommendations, and if so, whether the quality of the evidence justifies an endorsement. The Department of Health and Human Services and the Department of Agriculture together publish the recommendations as the "Dietary Guidelines for Americans" (http://www.health.gov/dietaryguidelines/dga2005/report/default.htm). Following their guidelines helps prevent the development of obesity, high blood pressure, and diabetes. The evidence also suggests, although with lesser certainty, that the recommendations might lower the risk of dementia, degenerative joint disease, and certain forms of cancer, particularly breast, ovarian, and colon cancer.

Dietary Guidelines for Americans 2005

- Limiting calories to the amount needed to maintain ideal weight
- Substituting mono- and polyunsaturated fats for saturated fats
- Emphasizing fruits, vegetables, and whole grains
- Decreasing intake of breads, pasta, cereals, and rice
- Eliminating refined sugars
- Limiting sodium intake
- Engaging in daily vigorous exercise

1 Please see the appendix for the Dietary Guidelines Advisory Committee membership.

During the last half of the twentieth century, some Americans had adopted better health habits, and the Center for Disease Control and Prevention reported a temporary decline in the number of deaths from cardiovascular disease (Ford, S. 2007, 2388). One of the reasons for the improvement was that some motivated people participated in fitness programs and avoided high-calorie foods containing saturated fat. Many quit smoking, so that only about 21 percent of American adults are smokers today, down from about 32 percent in the middle of the twentieth century.

Unfortunately, obesity has been replacing smoking as a more prevalent health hazard and improvement in longevity has slowed. Some experts predict that life expectancy might even begin to decline as a result (Bibbins-Domingo 2007, 2371). Recent data from the World Health Organization shows that the United States ranks only twenty-fourth among large industrialized nations in disability-adjusted life expectancy (Mathers 2000, 51).[2] We Americans have become overfed, oversized, and overconfident.

*The Hundred-Year Diet* has the overarching objective of encouraging real changes in health habits by first understanding the nature of the specific risks inherent in the typical American diet and sedentary life style. The next section identifies the most common degenerative diseases that cause early disability and death, and so their prevention becomes the target for measuring success. We highlight the research studies that demonstrate which changes in health habits result in predictable improved health outcomes. While no one can guarantee good health, every person can adopt those preventive steps known to reduce the risk of serious degenerative diseases. Aligning our health habits with recommendations proven to produce measurable benefits offers us our best chance. For example, we know that nonsmokers are much less likely than smokers to become respiratory cripples dragging along a portable oxygen tank. By not smoking, we can't guarantee ourselves immunity from emphysema, but our risk becomes infinitely small. The same logic applies to using nutrition and exercise in the prevention of heart disease, strokes, and diabetes.

For those who can make the change to a more prudent diet and regular vigorous exercise, feeling better and having an enhanced self-esteem become the immediate

2 Some authors have mistakenly assumed that inner-city violence underlies the poor longevity in the United States. Although crime rates may be higher in the United States than in some other countries where there is a longer life expectancy, the total number of American homicides was 17,694 during 2005, only about 0.7 percent of the total deaths. Exclusion of homicides would not have changed the disappointing life expectancy comparisons. Analyses of the data show that the higher prevalence of degenerative diseases causes the shorter life expectancy in the United States (National Vital Statistics Reports 2007).

rewards. Observe friends who are lean and physically active. Very likely they smile more and seem to enjoy life in contrast to sedentary people who often appear depressed. An exercise regimen often improves mood better than antidepressant drugs, as shown in several randomized clinical trials (Unützer 2007, 2271). Lean and energetic middle-aged people tend to remain lean and energetic as they age, and they more often avoid infirmity in their older years, too. My lean ninety-seven-year-old uncle chops wood every day and likes to tell jokes.

The next section lists the most common debilitating illnesses so that we can identify the highest priority targets for prevention. By knowing which diseases are most common, we can decide which preventive health habits will likely yield the most benefit. We should pay the closest attention to those recommendations that produce major reductions in the risk of common diseases, and worry less about doubtful speculations concerning causes of rare illnesses.

# *We Can Prevent Most Causes of Early Disability and Death.*

***Key Points***

- *Prevention works.*
- *Treatment is limited.*

Of the ten leading causes of disability and death in the United States, all are preventable to a significant degree with the possible exception of Alzheimer's disease. My medical practice of more than thirty years has taught me, that in spite of my patients' undaunted faith in the miracles of modern medicine, the benefits of medical treatment are really quite limited. Most of the patients treated in critical-care units survive to leave the hospital, but nearly all ultimately have a shorter-than-average life expectancy because of chronic illnesses. Medical care improves their symptoms and increases their functional capacity, but no one can restore completely the vigor that healthy people enjoy and take for granted.

The chart below lists the top ten causes of death according to the National Vital Statistics Reports published in 2007. Heart disease and strokes account for 32.4 percent of all deaths in both men and women, and significantly reduce the quality of life for survivors. Both diseases occur much less frequently in people who practice good health habits; however, both develop early and often in populations with a high incidence of obesity, high blood pressure, diabetes, and smoking. The major culprit is atherosclerosis, the deposit of plaques containing cholesterol and calcium in the lining of vital arteries. Prevention is effective, while treatment for heart disease and strokes has had only limited success. For example, the mortality rate for heart attacks is 30 percent, and more than half of the fatalities occur before the victim reaches a hospital for emergency treatment (Antman and Braunwald 2001). A study from the Netherlands in 2007 showed that 40 percent of all first heart attack victims died before being admitted to a hospital (Koek 2007, 434–441).

| | Cause of Death 2005 | Number |
|---|---|---|
| 1 | Heart disease | 649,399 |
| 2 | Cancer | 559,300 |
| 3 | Strokes | 143,397 |
| 4 | Emphysema | 130,957 |
| 5 | Accidents | 114,876 |
| 6 | Diabetes mellitus | 74,817 |
| 7 | Alzheimer's disease | 71,696 |
| 8 | Influenza and pneumonia | 62,804 |
| 9 | Kidney failure | 43,679 |
| 10 | Septicemia | 34,142 |

**Heart surgery limitations.** Numerous studies show that, although open-heart surgery[3] or coronary angioplasty[4] often relieve recurrent chest pain and other symptoms, patients who receive medication alone survive just as long, except in a few specific circumstances like multi-vessel disease. In a large study comparing survival rates following hospitalization for heart attacks, patients in Boston were eight times more likely than those in Toronto to undergo either open-heart surgery or coronary angioplasty. However, the investigators noted that "the one-year mortality rates were virtually identical (34.3 percent in the United States vs. 34.4 percent in Ontario)" (Tu 1997, 1500). Another investigator wrote that, although angioplasty and coronary bypass surgery are effective in relieving angina, "these procedures do not reduce mortality or the incidence of myocardial infarction compared to anti-anginal drugs" (Thadani 2004, S11–29). Heart surgery and angioplasty occasionally save lives in the short term, but they provide no guarantee against future heart attacks. A clot can form at any roughened area of atherosclerosis, even though the vessel is

3 Open heart surgery. Today, the most common form of open heart surgery is called a coronary artery bypass graft. Surgeons harvest a strip of vein from the leg and transplant it onto a coronary artery in the heart, bypassing a narrowed section.

4 Coronary angioplasty. Cardiologists use the term percutaneous coronary intervention (PCI) to mean balloon angioplasty or other catheterization techniques that open blocked coronary arteries. They pass the angioplasty catheter through a tiny incision in the skin into a major artery, usually in the thigh, and then thread the catheter up into a coronary artery in the heart. The operator then places the catheter tip into a targeted narrowed section of a coronary artery and inflates the balloon to widen the passage. Primary coronary angioplasty refers to an emergency procedure during a heart attack. Cardiologists often perform elective coronary angioplasty to relieve angina pectoris (chest pain).

only minimally narrowed, so patients following heart surgery or angioplasty are still at risk for heart attacks.

During the mid-1990s, more than five hundred thousand open heart operations per year were performed in the United States, but when surgeons discovered that overall survival had not improved, they became more selective, and the number of operations declined. Recent articles raise similar questions about a possible excessive use of angioplasty and stents,[5] especially for elective procedures to relieve angina pectoris (chest pain) (Kereiakes 2007, 1598–1603).

On the other hand, observations from long-term studies, like the one on the residents of Framingham, Massachusetts, show a marked reduction in the incidence of heart attacks and strokes in people who practice good health habits. They also suffer far less long-term physical or mental disability (Sytkowski 1990, 1635). In a recent clinical trial called the West of Scotland Coronary Prevention Study, diet and medication lowered cholesterol and reduced heart attacks by 30 percent in 6,345 men over a period of just five years (Ford, I 2007, 1477). Preventing heart disease before it has a chance to inflict permanent damage can make a huge difference in quality of life, while treatment after a portion of heart muscle has died can only help reduce the misery.

**Stroke treatment limitations.** Many medical centers promote early emergency treatment of strokes, but early treatment requires that a patient arrives within three hours after the onset of an acute stroke. In most communities, only a small percentage of acute stroke victims arrive before the deadline. Victims may not realize that their symptoms dictate urgency for treatment, or sometimes a victim is physically unable to call for help. Even those who arrive in an emergency department within three hours do not always receive treatment because the treatment itself carries a high risk and can be fatal. For example, clot-dissolving drugs used to reopen a blocked artery can themselves trigger intracranial bleeding, especially when certain risk factors are present such as high blood pressure, a common situation in acute stroke victims (Van der Worp 2007, 572-578). Nationwide, less than 1 percent of acute stroke victims ever receive clot-dissolving drugs. Practicing good health habits produces unlimited benefits in promoting a vigorous and active life contrasted with the stark limitations of treatment.

Neurologists advise early detection of patients who are at high risk for strokes and may recommend preventive surgery that offers some hope, but surgery also entails risk. The most common procedure, called a carotid endarterectomy,

---

5 Stents are small sleeves, often made of mesh, that cardiologists place in a coronary artery after expanding a narrowed area with a balloon catheter. They use stents to prevent recurrent narrowing of the coronary artery in the same place. Some stents contain medication to prevent clot formation.

opens a narrowed artery leading to the brain. Surgery and diagnostic angiograms can themselves cause a stroke or death, so strict guidelines limit these procedures to symptomatic patients at highest risk (U.S. Preventive Services Task Force 2007). For others, the risk exceeds the potential benefit. Just as with coronary heart disease, a clot can form at any location in a diseased carotid artery, and so successful surgery does not guarantee prevention of an acute stroke. Good health habits help evade the game of surgical roulette.

**Diabetes treatment limitations**. Diabetes mellitus has spread to affect more than 8 percent of the United States population and now ranks as the sixth-leading cause of death (National Vital Statistics Reports 2005). Type II diabetes accounts for more than 90 percent of all cases and is most often a complication of obesity, and thus often preventable. Obesity causes diabetes by increasing resistance to insulin, which normally acts on cell membranes to facilitate the transfer, metabolism, and storage of sugar. At the same time, diabetics develop a specific type of small blood vessel disease, which in combination with their higher prevalence of atherosclerosis in large vessels, leads to a greater potential for heart attacks and strokes. Diabetics also have a lesser chance for survival if a heart attack or stroke occurs. Vascular disease in diabetics causes many other problems too, such as blindness, kidney failure, and blockage of blood vessels leading to the legs. Treatment of type II diabetes with medication may improve blood sugar levels, but diabetics remain at high risk for vascular disease. If an overweight person with type II diabetes loses weight, insulin resistance diminishes and blood sugar levels improve. If weight loss is substantial, blood sugar levels may even become normal. In overweight diabetics, weight reduction is far more effective than medication.

**Other preventable diseases**. Of course, some preventable causes of death are unrelated to diet, such as emphysema, motor vehicle accidents, and influenza. We can all get a yearly flu vaccine, choose not to smoke, fasten our seat belts, and drive safely. Some of the more common types of cancer are partially preventable, too. Below are the predicted numbers of cancer deaths for 2007, as reported by the American Cancer Society, for the five most common causes of cancer deaths:

| Type of cancer | Number of Deaths |
|---|---|
| Lung | 160,000 |
| Colon | 52,000 |
| Breast | 40,000 |
| Pancreas | 33,000 |
| Prostate | 27,000 |

Lung cancer is the most common cause of cancer deaths, but it rarely occurs in nonsmokers, and so it is nearly 100 percent preventable. Colonoscopies at appropriate intervals can sharply reduce colon and rectal cancer deaths by removing polyps, which are known precursors of colon cancer. Some gastroenterologists and oncologists predict that pending long-term studies will show polyp removal to prevent as many as 50 percent of colon cancer deaths. Although some details about regular mammograms remain controversial, the American Cancer Society notes that a well-controlled trial in Sweden showed a 30 percent mortality reduction in breast cancer in patients screened with mammograms contrasted with those who were not (Duffy 2002, 451–457). Unfortunately, breast cancer deaths have declined only about 10 percent in the United States, related in part to a failure in achieving 100 percent screening. The mortality rate from prostate cancer has steadily declined since 1999, probably because of earlier detection and treatment (Walsh 2007, 2696). Prevention significantly reduces the mortality rate in four of the five most common types of cancer, lung, colon, breast, and prostate, which together cause nearly half of all cancer deaths. Even so, complacency and inertia in taking preventive steps trump the fear of developing cancer for many people.

**An ounce of prevention is worth a pound of cure.** History shows us that prevention is effective. In the first half of the twentieth century, life expectancy increased in the United States from 47.3 to 68.2 years between 1900 and 1950, a bonus of 20.9 years longer life. Modern medical treatment had not yet arrived by 1950. For example, 99 percent of the currently available drugs had not yet appeared—the first antibiotics did not become available until just before 1950—and intensive care units and modern surgical procedures like heart surgery were still on the horizon. Almost all of the increase in longevity in the first half of the twentieth century was due to prevention, such as the use of quarantine for infectious diseases like tuberculosis, the proliferation of immunizations, the introduction of clean water and sewage treatment, wider use of disinfectants and soap, the availability of refrigeration, and many other public health improvements that we take for granted today.

Since 1950, life expectancy has risen only an additional 9.7 years to 77.9 years in 2006. Although modern medical treatment has saved many lives, the surprisingly small longevity increase suggests that we have forgotten about prevention, especially the prevention of degenerative diseases. We sometimes expect that modern medicine can cure anything. In fact the treatment of heart disease, diabetes, and strokes is mostly palliative. For most degenerative diseases, we can improve symptoms, but rarely can we prevent disability and extend longevity. Through better health habits, such as attention to better nutrition and more exercise, we could all be trimmer, feel better, and enjoy a lifespan that could reach or exceed one hundred years. The next section describes how to evaluate the risk of degenerative diseases based on height and weight and to begin making some changes.

# *Obesity is a High-Risk, but Curable Disease.*

***Key Points***

- *Obesity disables and kills.*
- *Calories and exercise matter.*
- *The key to dieting is consistency.*

The spread of obesity is the number one serious public health problem in the United States. The Center for Disease Control and Prevention reports that 66 percent of American adults are overweight, defined as a body mass index (BMI) greater than twenty-five. Even worse, 31 percent of adults have a BMI greater than thirty, the threshold for a diagnosis of obesity. The extra weight promotes the development of cardiovascular disease by causing high blood pressure, cholesterol abnormalities, and diabetes mellitus, type II. Doctors call this combination the "metabolic syndrome," a cardiovascular time bomb.

For those persons who have a need to lose weight, the chart below may be helpful for planning purposes. The shaded part shows the range for a normal BMI and denotes an ideal weight. People who have a BMI above twenty-five, shown in the upper right-hand corner of the chart, run a greater risk of developing diabetes, high blood pressure, and cardiovascular disease. According to the chart, a person sixty-seven inches tall who weighs 190 pounds has a BMI of thirty, and would need to lose weight down to 160 pounds to attain a BMI of twenty-five in the ideal range. Likewise, a person whose BMI is already twenty-five should avoid gaining weight, since any increase would result in a BMI in the overweight range.

Body Mass Index (BMI)
BMI = 703 × Weight (lb)/ $\text{Height}^2$ ($\text{in}^2$)
Normal = 20 to 25
(Slightly lower for children and older adults)

| height (inches) | weight (pounds) | | | | | | | | | | | |
|---|---|---|---|---|---|---|---|---|---|---|---|---|
| | ***120*** | ***130*** | ***140*** | ***150*** | ***160*** | ***170*** | ***180*** | ***190*** | ***200*** | ***210*** | ***220*** | ***230*** |
| ***60*** | 23 | 25 | 27 | 29 | 31 | 33 | 35 | 37 | 39 | 41 | 42 | 43 |
| ***61*** | 23 | 25 | 27 | 28 | 30 | 32 | 34 | 36 | 38 | 40 | 40 | 42 |
| ***62*** | 22 | 24 | 26 | 27 | 29 | 31 | 33 | 35 | 37 | 38 | 39 | 40 |
| ***63*** | 21 | 23 | 25 | 27 | 28 | 30 | 32 | 34 | 36 | 37 | 38 | 39 |
| ***64*** | 21 | 22 | 24 | 26 | 28 | 29 | 31 | 33 | 34 | 36 | 37 | 38 |
| ***65*** | 20 | 22 | 23 | 25 | 27 | 28 | 30 | 32 | 33 | 35 | 36 | 37 |
| ***66*** | 19 | 21 | 23 | 24 | 26 | 27 | 29 | 31 | 32 | 34 | 35 | 36 |
| ***67*** | 19 | 20 | 22 | 24 | 25 | 27 | 28 | 30 | 31 | 33 | 34 | 35 |
| ***68*** | 18 | 20 | 21 | 23 | 24 | 26 | 27 | 29 | 30 | 32 | 33 | 34 |
| ***69*** | 18 | 19 | 21 | 22 | 24 | 25 | 27 | 28 | 30 | 31 | 32 | 33 |
| ***70*** | 17 | 19 | 20 | 22 | 23 | 24 | 26 | 27 | 29 | 30 | 31 | 32 |
| ***71*** | 17 | 18 | 20 | 21 | 22 | 24 | 25 | 27 | 28 | 29 | 30 | 31 |
| ***72*** | 16 | 18 | 19 | 20 | 22 | 23 | 24 | 26 | 27 | 28 | 29 | 30 |
| ***73*** | 16 | 17 | 19 | 20 | 21 | 22 | 24 | 25 | 26 | 28 | 28 | 29 |
| ***74*** | 15 | 17 | 18 | 19 | 21 | 22 | 23 | 24 | 25 | 27 | 28 | 28 |
| ***75*** | 15 | 16 | 18 | 19 | 20 | 21 | 23 | 24 | 25 | 26 | 27 | 28 |

**Is thinner better?** A BMI below twenty sometimes indicates serious chronic disease, but more often a low BMI is just a variation of normal, especially in children and the elderly. Chronic illnesses are usually evident long before the BMI declines; consequently a person who has a low BMI, but no apparent illness, probably has an excellent life expectancy. Normal children typically have a BMI lower than that of adults. Older adults should have a lower BMI than younger adults because of less bone and muscle mass. Ideally, the BMI later in life should be no more than it was at age twenty.

Some researchers have noted that long-term caloric restriction reduces age-related diseases and extends life span in other species. For example, mice fed a calorie-restricted diet live longer than those from the same litter that are fed normally. Long-term observations of the high prevalence of centenarians in Okinawa have given credibility to the argument that caloric restriction in humans may extend life as it does in mice. Elderly Okinawans typically have had a lifelong low BMI and enjoy an extended mean and maximum life span (Willcox 2007, 434–455).

However, a study from Harvard examining the metabolic differences between mouse and human systems predicts that, "the large increases in mean life span and maximum life-span potential observed in laboratory rodents subject to caloric restriction will not obtain in human populations." The analysis further predicts that caloric restriction will have a "relatively minor effect on the mean life span of non-obese populations" (Demetrius 2006, 66–82). Nevertheless, we should not dismiss the observations of the long life span of lean Okinawans, recognizing that real-life experiences do not always reflect theoretical projections.

**Childhood obesity on the rise**. Recently, the incidence of childhood obesity has mushroomed so that one in every three children is either overweight or obese (Ogden 2006, 1549). For several years, the Center for Disease Control and Prevention has been warning that children born today will have a shorter life expectancy than their parents as a result of the obesity epidemic (Olshansky 2005, 1138). A recent review of health records of 276,835 Danish children born between 1930 and 1976 showed that children even minimally overweight risked heart attacks later in life. Researchers observed that children only ten pounds overweight had a measurable increase in the risk of cardiovascular disease, and those whose BMI was in the obese range later suffered a very high incidence of heart attacks. For example, a thirteen-year-old boy whose weight is twenty-three pounds above the ideal BMI has a "33 percent increase in the probability of his having a coronary heart disease event before the age of 60" (Baker 2007, 2329).

Children in the United States today are more overweight than those in the Danish study, so predictions of shorter life expectancy and disabling adult illnesses are even worse than the experience in Denmark would indicate (Ludwig 2007, 2325). Statisticians are now warning that by the year 2035, the incidence of coronary heart disease will have increased to more than one hundred thousand excess cases attributable to increased obesity among today's adolescents (Bibbins-Domingo 2007, 2371). Obese children suffer a long list of complications that continue into their adult life.

**Complications of Childhood Obesity, partial list**

| | |
|---|---|
| Psychological | Poor self-esteem<br>Social isolation<br>Anxiety and Depression |
| Metabolic | Insulin resistance<br>Type II diabetes mellitus<br>Cholesterol abnormalities |
| Cardiovascular | High blood pressure<br>Exercise intolerance |
| Pulmonary | Sleep apnea<br>Asthma |
| Gastrointestinal | Gallstones<br>Gastroesophageal reflux<br>Fatty liver |
| Renal | Glomerulosclerosis |
| Musculoskeletal | Slipped growth center<br>Back pain |

From Ludwig, David S. 2007. *New England Journal of Medicine*. 357 (23), 2325.

**Friends influence eating habits.** A recent *New England Journal of Medicine* report of 12,067 participants in the Framingham Heart Study in Massachusetts demonstrated that obesity spreads through social ties more than as a result of heredity. Researchers observed that a person's chances of becoming obese increased by 57 percent if a close friend became obese at the same time. Obesity was also more likely if siblings or a spouse became obese, but casual acquaintances had no measurable influence on body weight (Christakis 2007, 370). Obesity develops as a result of bad habits that we learn from each other; our best friends may be bad for our health.

One of my patients observed this phenomenon during her experiences in a community theater where a charismatic, lean, energetic director influenced the behavior of the actors. The director had been a dancer and was physically animated as he coached and encouraged the members of the cast. During the course of rehearsals and performances, nearly all of the actors tried to be like the director, and so most lost weight. In other plays in the same theater group, but with a more sedentary director, the energy level of a different cast lagged. Actors selected for roles tended to be overweight. The sedentary director invited the cast members to go out with him for midnight dessert after the rehearsals and performances, an offer most cast members enthusiastically accepted. The actors admired both directors and subconsciously followed the physical activity and eating-habit norms set by them.

**The snack problem**. Anything packaged in cellophane and decorated in four colors is probably a poor nutrition choice. Treats have become an everyday self-reward, as ice cream, candy bars, and cookies have displaced fresh fruit in schools, offices, and on soccer fields. Television advertising effectively manipulates behavior by encouraging snacking and promoting the sale of profitable high-calorie, high-fat, and high-sugar-containing products. Nearly one quarter of all television advertisements promotes eating, but rarely are fresh fruits and vegetables on the menu. Eating while watching television prompts mindless, mechanical munching encouraged by the television monitor. We can counter all of this by turning off the television set, eliminating snacking, and returning to planned meals with family and friends. Successful weight control begins with a return to good eating habits.

**The supersize problem**. Large portion size often defeats those who have difficulty maintaining an ideal weight. For those who want to include red meat in their diet, many nutrition experts explain that a three-ounce portion equals the size of a deck of cards, more than enough for anyone, including elementary school-aged children. Consider that vegetarians consume adequate amounts of protein from non-meat sources such as beans, seeds, and nuts. Restaurants often serve eight-, ten-, and even twelve-ounce portions of red meat that some people think of as normal. A ten-ounce steak has seven hundred to nine hundred calories. A McDonald's Double Quarter Pounder with cheese has 740 calories, and a large-sized portion of French fries (six ounces) has 570 calories. Burger King's Double Cheeseburger with bacon has five hundred calories, and a chocolate shake has 660 (Pennington 1998, 110, 116, and 118). Many restaurants publish charts online that show the calories and fat content of the items on their menu. Regular customers should familiarize themselves with this important information.

**Calories matter.** Any diet can result in weight reduction, as long as the calories consumed do not exceed the amount needed to maintain an ideal weight. Two recent studies, one from Stanford University (Dansinger 2005, 43-53) and one from Israel (Shai 2008, 229-41), showed that whether a diet is carbohydrate-restricted or fat-restricted is irrelevant (Dansinger 2005, 43

–53). The laws of thermodynamics regulate a person's weight; weight loss occurs when there is a combination of increased exercise and caloric restriction. The reduced fat in *The Hundred-Year Diet* recipes aid in weight control, as one gram of fat contains nine calories, while one gram of carbohydrate or protein has only four. However, most people who want to lose weight will still find that a consistent commitment to dietary restraint is unavoidable for success. Most dieters can reorient toward better eating habits by paying close attention to the quality and quantity of various foods, and then planning and adhering to daily menus. Consistency helps to develop proper nutrition as a long-term habit. The following first steps can help:

- Eliminating splurging: We change our eating habits only with a sense of loss and depression. High-fat, high-sugar, and high-calorie foods are our favorites, and giving them up can generate peer pressure and ridicule: "What harm can one little piece of chocolate cake do?" Celebrating special occasions by consuming high-calorie food "just this one time" usually evolves into a bad habit. Celebrate instead with a physically active event or by attaining a new exercise milestone.
- Measuring portions: Gaining experience by weighing and measuring portions for a few days helps one to learn how to estimate smaller quantities.
- Emphasizing raw and steamed vegetables: Portion size is less important for fresh fruit and vegetables. An apple has only about eighty calories and an orange has sixty. A cup of steamed spinach or zucchini has less than twenty calories and a raw tomato has only about twenty-five. Have a second helping.
- Keeping a journal: We can learn a lot about ourselves by creating daily menus and keeping a food journal to reacclimatize to the desired variety and quantity of food.
- Weighing daily: Everyone needs feedback to measure progress, and bathroom scales give an honest and impartial assessment.
- Reading labels: Rice and sugar constitute the main ingredients of a popular, widely advertised breakfast cereal promoted as an aid to weight reduction. The suggested nonfat milk and fruit topping contain all of the claimed nutritional benefit. Read the labels.
- Passing up eating on the run: Eating while working, walking, or driving is mindless and leads to weight gain. The cup holder may pose more danger to drivers of motor vehicles than any defective part subject to recall. Try to eat only at planned mealtimes with family or friends.

- Skipping the power lunch: Restaurants and cafeterias serve high-calorie, high-fat foods. Brown bag it instead. Some options that help comply with the USDA nutritional guidelines are:

| **Brown Bag Ideas** |
|---|
| fruit, both fresh and dried |
| crudités (carrots, celery, bell pepper, cherry tomatoes) |
| unsalted nuts (small quantities) |
| whole wheat seeded bagel or bread slice |
| low-fat, low-sodium rye crackers |
| hard-boiled eggs (skip the yolk) |
| nonfat yogurt or cottage cheese |
| peanut butter or hummus (small quantities) |

Controlling the amount of fat in the diet helps to reduce calories, because fats have more than twice as many calories as carbohydrates or proteins; and emphasizing a reduction in intake of saturated fat and trans fat not only helps control weight, but also improves blood cholesterol levels.

# *Every Body Deserves a Normal Cholesterol.*

***Key Points***

- *Trans fats and saturated fats raise harmful LDL cholesterol.*[6]
- *Unsaturated fats like olive oil lower LDL cholesterol.*

Abnormal blood levels of cholesterol and triglycerides cause more than half of the heart disease in the United States. Cholesterol and triglycerides are fats, also called lipids, which circulate in the blood as part of a transport system for storage of nutrients. In the bloodstream, proteins attach to lipids to form lipoproteins, large molecules that can travel easily to and from fat cells. Although gene defects produce some lipoprotein abnormalities, most often we cause the problem ourselves with a diet high in saturated fat, a sedentary lifestyle, and excess weight. Below are normal lipoprotein blood levels as published in Harrison's *Principles of Internal Medicine*. A high LDL, which transports cholesterol, correlates strongly with the risk of heart disease. Elevation of VLDL, consisting mostly of triglycerides, carries a moderate risk. HDL protects against heart disease, so higher is better (Ginsberg 2001, Chapter 344).

| Laboratory Test | Normal |
|---|---|
| Total Cholesterol | <200 mg/dl[7] |
| LDL (low density lipoprotein, mostly cholesterol) | <130 mg/dl |
| VLDL (very low density lipoproteins, mostly triglycerides) | <150 mg/dl |
| HDL (high density lipoprotein) | >40 mg/dl (men)<br>>50 mg/dl (women) |

6 Please see the Appendix for a further explanation of the terms triglycerides, saturated fat, unsaturated fat, trans fat, LDL, VLDL, HDL.

7 Laboratories must measure the total cholesterol in order to compute the other lipoprotein values, but the total cholesterol itself is less important than the LDL, VLDL, and HDL for diagnostic purposes.

People who already have heart disease or diabetes should aim for an even lower LDL level and a higher HDL than above. In some Asian countries, observed average lipid levels are better than the normal levels above, and as a consequence, some professional medical organizations now recommend lower targets for LDL, even for primary prevention in normal people with no evidence of cardiovascular disease. Anyone who desires to improve cholesterol levels by means of a diet should consistently avoid consuming saturated fat and trans fat, because intermittent or insufficient restriction may not yield any measurable difference. Strict avoidance of the harmful forms of dietary fat reduces LDL by about 15 percent in most people, a major improvement of an important risk factor associated with cardiovascular disease.

Just following the recommendations of the Dietary Guidelines for Americans should result in normal blood lipid levels for most people. Others should ask about adding a cholesterol-lowering drug to reach an optimal cholesterol profile (Domanski 2007, 1543). Use drugs only as an aid to dietary control of cholesterol, never as a rationalization for dietary indiscretion. Drugs have occasional serious side effects, even those approved by the Food and Drug Administration; consequently, physicians try to administer the fewest number of drugs at the lowest possible dose that will still attain important measurable objectives.

**Avoid trans fat.** Commercial food processing sometimes converts unsaturated vegetable oil into partially-hydrogenated trans fat. Many restaurants prefer using trans fat for deep-frying because of its stability at high temperatures and minimal smoke emission. Trans fats are more solid at room temperature, a characteristic that eliminates greasy stains on packages of cookies, crackers, and chips, and thus improves their attractiveness on store shelves. If more healthful liquid oils were used, snacks would taste, feel, and appear greasy. Bakery goods made with trans fat also have a longer shelf life than those made with liquid oils, a convenience for both food markets and consumers. Bakers prefer trans fat for pie shells, puff pastry, and the icing on cakes to make their desserts seem lighter and less greasy. Cakes with icing made with trans fat appear freshly-made for days. Appearances deceive; always read the labels (Mozaffarian 2006, 1601–1613).

Avoid the following:

- Vegetable oil labeled as trans fat or partially-hydrogenated
- Most deep-fried foods, such as French fries, chips, or fried chicken
- Palm oil, coconut oil, and cocoa butter
- Dairy fat, such as butter, cream, ice cream, cheese, whole milk
- Stick margarine
- Animal fat, except for fish

**Avoid saturated fat, too.** Although some restaurants and food markets have begun to eliminate foods containing trans fat, many consumers have become complacent about saturated fat, which can cause atherosclerosis just like processed trans fat. Almost 70 percent of the fat in cream is already saturated, so that butter, ice cream, and cheese worsen cholesterol blood levels, too. Butter is no better than stick margarine. Red meat and cocoa butter are other examples of foods high in saturated fat. Often the food served in elegant and expensive restaurants contains as much harmful fat as that served in fast-food outlets, so that high-priced chefs are no guarantee that their creations will be healthful. They aim to please your palate, not your coronary arteries.

### Examples of Saturated Fat Calories

| | *Percent Fat* | *Percent of total fat that is Saturated* |
|---|---|---|
| High Saturated Fat | | |
| Butter | 100% | 64% |
| Ice cream | 60% | 61% |
| Blue cheese | 73% | 65% |
| Beef steak | 66% | 40% |
| Baker's chocolate | 62% | 62% |
| Low Saturated Fat | | |
| Olive oil | 100% | 9% |
| Olives | 72% | 5% |
| Salmon | 30% | 12% |
| Almonds | 79% | 8% |
| Macadamia nuts | 95% | 5% |

**Use unsaturated fats.** Many studies have shown that certain types of fat in the diet actually improve cholesterol levels. Replacing saturated fats and trans fats with monounsaturated fatty acids, found in olive oil, can produce another 10 to 15 percent reduction in harmful LDL levels beyond that achievable with just fat restriction alone. Fish oil contains large amounts of omega-3 fatty acids, which may provide some protection against the development of cardiovascular disease. Many plant foods and polyunsaturated oils, such as corn, safflower, or canola oil, contain omega-6 fatty acids that may be beneficial, too (Lemaitre 2003, 319–325).[8] Older studies suggest that a high ratio of omega-6 fatty acids to omega-3 fatty acids may be harmful, but recent studies from Harvard conclude: "Adequate intake of both omega-6

8 Please see the section on nutritional supplements for an analysis of the current status of fish oil and omega-3 and omega-6 fatty acids as dietary supplements.

and omega-3 fatty acids are essential for good health and low rates of cardiovascular disease and type II diabetes, but the ratio of these fatty acids is not useful" (Willett 2007, S42–45 and Mozaffarian 2005, 157–164). All of the recipes in The Hundred-Year Diet are low in calories, saturated fat, and cholesterol, while assuring a moderate amount of monounsaturated vegetable oil, omega-3, and omega-6 fatty acids. None have any trans fat.

Recommended Mono- and Polyunsaturated Fats

- Olives and olive oil
- Fish and fish oil
- Corn, safflower, and Canola oils
- Seeds and nuts

**HDL protects against heart disease.** HDL is a cholesterol-containing lipoprotein that protects against the development of atherosclerosis. Recent studies have shown that abnormally low HDL blood levels predict heart attacks and strokes more reliably than the other lipid measurements. Even patients who have achieved ideal LDL or VLDL levels by means of diet and/or medication are at considerable risk if the HDL is too low (Barter 2007, 1301). People who are obese, have elevated VLDL levels, or are diabetic are more likely to have a low HDL than others. Weight reduction will yield some improvement, but diet alone is often insufficient. Medication is almost always recommended. Any person with a low HDL, or any other significant cholesterol abnormality, should consult a physician.

**Ideal dietary fat content.** In the typical American diet, more than 35 percent of the calories come from fat, and for many people the percentage exceeds 50 percent, especially for those who are lovers of butter, ice cream, French fries, and red meat. The National Cholesterol Education Program (www.nhlbi.nih.gov/chd/) recommends the following diet composition:

| | |
|---|---|
| Total fat | <30% |
| Fatty Acids | |
| Saturated | <7% |
| Polyunsaturated | <10% |
| Monounsaturated | 10–15% |
| Carbohydrate | 50–60% |
| Protein | 10–20% |
| Cholesterol | <200 mg/day |

Some researchers, such as the Dietary Approaches to Stop Hypertension (DASH) Collaborative Research Group cited in the next section, recommend that total fat be further restricted to less than 25 percent of the total. Please note on the chart above that 80 to 90 percent of the calories come from either fats or carbohydrates. Since most nutrition experts recommend limiting the amount of fat in the diet to no more than 25 or 30 percent, most of the rest must come from carbohydrates, preferably from fruits, vegetables, and whole grain sources. Nevertheless, some weight-reduction diets promote restricting carbohydrates, which means that a higher proportion of calories must come from fat. "Low carb" is just another way of saying "high fat." Physicians consider consuming large amounts of fat long-term to be ill-advised because high fat diets are one of the causes of atherosclerosis.

The reasoning behind the low carb movement comes from research during the 1950s and 1960s. Both fats and carbohydrates are sources of energy, but carbohydrates are an immediate source, while fats must go through a complex metabolic process before they can be used for energy. The conversion itself requires energy that must come from glucose, a carbohydrate. If we limit carbohydrates in the diet, the conversion of fat becomes inefficient and results in remnants called ketoacids that circulate in the blood. We eliminate some ketoacids in the urine, thereby shedding calories, but the total reduction is only a few calories per day.

Some low carb advocates assert that ketoacids curb the appetite, and thus lead to weight loss; in fact, it is true that most people don't feel well with a high level of ketoacids in the blood. An extreme form can occur in type I diabetics who develop an emergency situation called ketoacidosis. So far, studies have failed to prove that ketogenic diets lead to persistent weight loss (Dansinger 2005, 43–53). Physicians warn that long-term, low carb diets can increase harmful forms of cholesterol, and that those dieters who elect to try them should restrict their use to brief periods of time. The Hundred-Year Diet strives to build good health habits that last, and so low carb diets play no role. Fruits, vegetables, and whole grain, high-fiber foods are nearly 100 percent carbohydrate, and they are not your enemy; these foods help lower your cholesterol and control your blood pressure, as we shall see in the next section.

# *The DASH Diet: Can Diet Alone Improve High Blood Pressure?*

***Key Points***

- *Sodium restriction below three thousand milligrams per day helps reduce blood pressure.*
- *Fruits and vegetables further reduce blood pressure.*
- *One teaspoon of salt equals 1,600 milligrams of sodium and four thousand milligrams of sodium chloride.*
- *High salt intake interferes with blood pressure medicine.*

In 1996, a large group of collaborating researchers introduced a new diet called DASH, Dietary Approaches to Stop Hypertension. The objective was to measure if a diet rich in fruits and vegetables, but low in saturated fat, would further reduce the blood pressure levels achievable with salt restriction alone. They maintained sodium levels at the recommended maximum of three thousand milligrams per day, but reduced fat to less than 25 percent of total calories, which were adjusted to maintain the same weight before and during the dietary restrictions. Significant additional reduction in blood pressure resulted in participants who used the DASH diet in contrast to those who used salt restriction alone (Appel 1997, 1117).

However, subsequent clinical trials where participants inconsistently followed the DASH diet showed no advantage. The researchers concluded that a high level of compliance with the DASH diet was required for measurable blood pressure reduction, similar to the conclusions about effectiveness in improving cholesterol levels through diet (Folsom 2007, 225). In 2005, the Dietary Guidelines Advisory Committee incorporated into their own recommendations the same conclusions of the DASH Collaborative Research Group: marked restriction of saturated fat, substituting fruits and vegetables for some of the bread portions, and limiting sodium intake to no more than three thousand milligrams per day.

For most people with high blood pressure, taking medication is necessary to prevent the high rate of heart disease and strokes that uncontrolled high blood pressure used to cause prior to the introduction of effective antihypertensive medicines in the middle of the twentieth century. However, reducing sodium (salt) in the diet is also an important part of treatment programs, but it is especially so for patients taking diuretics. Diuretics usually cause a reduction of potassium levels in the blood, which a diet high in sodium will accentuate to potentially dangerous levels. Many physicians prescribe potassium chloride as a substitute for table salt, not only to avoid sodium, but also to help maintain a normal potassium blood level. Sea salt and Kosher salt present the same high-sodium hazard as ordinary commercial table salt because they all contain sodium chloride. Most restaurant food also contains large amounts of sodium, far above the maximum daily recommendation of three thousand milligrams per day for anyone with high blood pressure. Some restaurant meals top ten thousand milligrams of sodium, and restaurant diners often notice increased thirst within an hour after an elegant restaurant meal, revealing that the chef likes to use plenty of salt. Elegant dining can sometimes resemble drinking seawater.

The DASH diet alone may not be sufficient for adequate control of high blood pressure in everyone, but adherence to the diet may improve the level of control, reduce the amount of medication needed, and avoid the risk of heart rhythm disturbances that a low blood level of potassium can cause. For those people who have only marginal elevation of blood pressure, following the DASH diet recommendations and losing weight might be all that they need for maintaining a normal blood pressure. The same dietary regimen should also improve blood lipoprotein measurements.

# *Does Sugar Promote Obesity? Do Whole Grains and Fiber Prevent it?*

***Key Points***

*High-fiber and whole grain foods may help:*

- *control weight.*
- *improve serum cholesterol.*
- *prevent colorectal disease including cancer.*

Human beings love sugar; just watch any infant who experiences his first taste. So why do the Dietary Guidelines for Americans recommend a marked reduction in the consumption of refined sugar and high-fructose corn syrup? And what's so important about whole grains and dietary fiber?

Reasons for eliminating refined sugar include the prevention of dental caries and the avoidance of foods that lack any nutritional value, except for the added calories. High-fructose corn syrup raises serum triglyceride levels (VLDL), although whether this is harmful to normal people remains uncertain (Brunzell 2007, 1009–1017). Some authors speculate that sugar also causes obesity, noting that the spread of obesity occurred at about the same time as the increased availability of sugar. They argue that sugar-containing foods stimulate the appetite in a way that overcomes normal satiety signals. Most acknowledge that other variables may also play an important role in promoting obesity, such as the rise in per capita income coupled with enhanced productivity and cheaper prices of food. Others assert that our high-stress, competitive culture fosters a compulsion for short-term self-reward in the form of sugar-containing snacks.

**Sugar may stimulate hunger.** Simple sugars cause a faster and higher spike in blood sugar than complex carbohydrates. After rapid ingestion of a simple sugar, such as in a soft drink, the blood sugar rises very quickly to a peak, sometimes in only about twenty minutes. Insulin reacts immediately, leading to an equally rapid fall in blood sugar to very low levels within another twenty or thirty minutes, stimulating hunger. In some people, the hunger symptoms are intense and accompanied by anxiety from the release of adrenalin in response to the low blood sugar. A low blood sugar also stimulates high levels of other hormones (cortisol and growth hormone) that tend to worsen wide swings in blood sugar levels. This high/low blood sugar cycle, called reactive hypoglycemia, does not signify diabetes or other underlying serious disease, but it can be uncomfortable. Some physicians speculate that recurrent mild reactive hypoglycemia from ingestion of simple sugars causes obesity by stirring hunger and encouraging people to snack throughout the day. No clinical studies exist to document the hypothesis, but the concept is reasonable enough.

**Some complex carbohydrates may modulate hunger.** Digestive enzymes convert complex carbohydrates rapidly into simple sugars in the gut, and so the blood sugar can rise quickly after ingestion of certain complex starches, too. However, most complex carbohydrates contain substances that inhibit the speed of assimilation and delay the rise in blood sugar. An example is pectin, a kind of soluble fiber in many vegetables and in the skin of many types of fruit. If we eat an apple with the skin, which contains pectin, the blood sugar rises more slowly than if we peel the apple first to remove the skin. Likewise, pectin stirred into plain sugar water and ingested will retard the rise in blood sugar. Most sugar-containing drinks and other sweet snacks do not contain pectin or other assimilation-inhibiting substances, and thus their consumption may induce a sense of hunger within an hour after ingestion. Replacing simple sugars with complex carbohydrates has special value for insulin-dependant diabetics to help modulate their blood sugar.

**High-fiber foods may prevent heart disease and cancer.** The Dietary Guidelines for Americans suggest replacing simple sugars with high-fiber and whole grain foods for other reasons as well. Some advocates point to countries where the populations consume high-fiber diets, and where the incidences of heart disease and colon cancer are low. However, other variables may play a role in those countries, such as a limited availability of red meat and other high-fat foods, a low prevalence of obesity, minimum use of tobacco and alcohol, and greater physical activity. Nevertheless, since the substitution of whole grains for simple sugars entails no risk, the speculation about the benefit is strong enough for the Dietary Guidelines Advisory Committee to justify making a recommendation in favor of a high fiber, whole grain diet.

**Soluble and Insoluble Fiber (Sizer 1994, 106)**

| | *Health Effects* | *Examples of Food Sources* |
|---|---|---|
| Soluble fiber | Slows sugar assimilation<br>Binds and eliminates some cholesterol<br>Promotes a sense of satiety | Fruit (oranges, grapes, etc.)<br>Beans (pinto, kidney, etc.)<br>Oats, oat bran<br>Rye<br>Seeds<br>Barley<br>Many vegetables |
| Insoluble fiber | Softens stool and prevents constipation<br>May prevent hemorrhoids, irritable bowel syndrome, and diverticulosis<br>May reduce colon cancer risk | Whole grains<br>Wheat bran<br>Brown rice<br>Seeds<br>Beans<br>Many vegetables |

Fiber in food comes in two types: soluble and insoluble, both of which increase the sense of satiety to dampen the urge to snack. Soluble fiber absorbs cholesterol like a sponge, but it is too large to be assimilated, and so the fiber and cholesterol together pass through the gut for elimination. How much cholesterol and saturated fat are removed by soluble fiber remains uncertain, and estimates vary greatly. The question is further complicated because high fiber foods contain little cholesterol or saturated fat; consequently, the improved serum cholesterol levels may relate more to reduced dietary fat intake than to greater removal by soluble fiber. Whether by reducing harmful fat in the diet, or by greater removal from the gut, high fiber foods improve the level of cholesterol in the blood.

Many foods also contain insoluble fiber, which absorbs water and swells slowing the movement of food in the upper intestine, creating a more durable sense of fullness. It then stimulates and distends the muscles of the lower digestive tract to maintain a normal tone and prevent constipation. Many gastroenterologists think that insoluble fiber helps prevent hemorrhoids, irritable bowel syndrome, and diverticulosis. Some scientists speculate that insoluble fiber prevents contact of cancer-causing chemicals with the lining of the colon by carrying toxins through the colon for elimination.

**Some Common High-Fiber Foods**

| | grams |
|---|---|
| Rye flour, 1 cup | 28.9 |
| Whole wheat flour, 1 cup | 14.6 |
| Black beans, boiled, 1 cup | 15.0 |
| Lima beans, boiled, 1 cup | 13.2 |
| Oatmeal, steel cut, dry, 1 cup | 16.0 |
| Acorn squash, baked, 1 cup | 9.0 |
| Green peas, 1 cup | 8.8 |
| Avocado, 1 medium | 8.5 |
| Blackberries, 1 cup | 7.6 |
| Apple, 1 whole with skin | 3.7 |
| Brown rice, cooked, 1 cup | 3.5 |

**Clinical trials show tentative support for high-fiber diets.** High-fiber and whole grain foods probably help prevent atherosclerosis and other diseases, but few clinical trials exist to document whether or not they are effective (Seal 2006, 24). Several clinical trials have demonstrated that whole grain oats improve serum cholesterol, and thus may prevent coronary heart disease, but unfortunately, other variables may have influenced the results. For example, participants who consumed more fiber might also have reduced saturated fat intake at the same time. Since high-fiber foods are generally low in total fat, but contain abundant amounts of beneficial omega-3 and omega-6 fatty acids, the dietary fat profile may have caused some or all of the observed serum cholesterol improvement.

All of the studies on high-fiber diets to date contain design flaws. Most were of very short duration, sometimes lasting only a few weeks, and rarely more than two years. Companies with commercial interests in whole grain foods funded many of the trials, and thus had a stake in demonstrating a beneficial outcome for high-fiber diets. Nevertheless, the consistent results of numerous clinical trials showed that participants who consumed oat bran had lower LDL and total cholesterol (Truswell 2002, 1). Whether whole grains other than oats have a similar benefit is less certain (Kelly 2007, CD005051).

Unfortunately, long-term, randomized clinical trials to assess the effectiveness of high-fiber diets in preventing disease have not been possible to date. Most people in the United States and Canada prefer a low-fiber, high-fat diet, and thus, enrolling large numbers of volunteers willing to endure dietary restrictions for experimental periods of several years has not been practical, as experienced in a recent Stanford University study (Dansinger 2005, 43–53).

Nevertheless, dietary factors as a possible cause of colorectal disease remain a serious concern, because there are significant differences in the incidence of various colorectal diseases in genetically similar populations. For example, the incidence of colon cancer is much higher in Japanese Americans than in Japanese nationals. Conversely, Japanese nationals have a higher incidence of stomach cancer than do their relatives living in the United States. Diet is the most obvious difference in the two populations, acknowledging that targeting a high-fat, low-fiber diet as the specific cause may be premature. Speculation about other dietary causes of colorectal disease includes red meat and alcohol, as well as deficiencies of folic acid, vitamin D, and calcium (Ryan-Harshman 2007, 1913).

For the moment, there is sufficient theoretical reason to support the recommendation to replace simple sugars with fruits, vegetables, and whole grain, high-fiber foods, and to moderate the intake of red meat and alcohol. Anyone with a snacking problem or any diabetic taking insulin should seriously consider eliminating simple sugars and substituting complex carbohydrates and whole grains. Estimates of the optimal amount of fiber needed range from twenty-five to forty grams per day, depending upon the daily calorie needs. Switching to a high-fiber, whole grain diet incurs no risk, and the benefits might be substantial.

# *What's in a Healthful Diet?*

*Key Points*

- *Limit calories.*
- *Emphasize fruits and vegetables.*
- *Replace processed grain with whole grains.*
- *Cancel the butter; use olive oil.*
- *Choose fish, chicken breasts, beans, and nuts.*

The Dietary Guidelines for Americans recommendations resemble the Mediterranean diet emerging in the 1950s from a study on the island of Crete, where the population appeared to have had a greater longevity than in northern European countries. Like the Dietary Guidelines for Americans, the original Mediterranean diet emphasized fruits, vegetables, and whole grain cereals. Olive oil replaced butter and cream; beans, fish, and poultry replaced red meat. Other risk factors unrelated to diet may also have played a role in producing the observed longer life span, such as more physical activity and less cigarette smoking. The people who lived on Crete often drank red wine, but so did their northern cousins, and thus, red wine consumption probably did not cause the observed greater longevity. The Mediterranean people who drank red wine also happened to have a more healthful diet and possessed more health-promoting habits then people who lived in northern European cities (Willett 1995, 1402S). Unfortunately, people living in Mediterranean countries today consume more calories and more saturated fat than in 1950; consequently, there is more obesity, and the incidence of heart disease now resembles that observed in northern European countries.

Since the 1950s, numerous studies on populations adhering to a diet like the one found on Crete have shown reduced mortality from heart disease and cancer. Recent studies point to avoidance of obesity and a higher ratio of unsaturated fats to saturated fats as the most important individual elements in the original Mediterranean diet that led to the increased longevity (Hu

2003, 2596). The current Dietary Guidelines for Americans emphasizes those elements.

**The Personal Diet Pyramid.** The U.S. Department of Agriculture supports a Web site for calculating a personal diet pyramid based on the Dietary Guidelines for Americans (www.mypyramid.gov). Each person should adjust the recommended nutritional guidelines for age, BMI, and level of physical activity. For instance, a person who engages in sixty minutes of vigorous daily exercise requires three hundred to five hundred calories per day more than a sedentary person to maintain the same weight. Someone whose BMI exceeds twenty-five will need to reduce calories below the maintenance level in order to lose weight. Older people usually require fewer calories than do young adults. Below is an average adult calorie pattern of two thousand calories, which must be adjusted according to each individual's needs. Please note that most people do not need to restrict certain raw or steamed vegetables to the recommended quantities. An extra serving or two of lettuce, celery, or spinach will make almost no difference in the day's total calorie count.

**2000 Calorie Diet by Food Groups**

| *Food Group* | *Quantity* |
|---|---|
| Grains<br>5 ounces | Limit to five slices of bread or equivalent amount of cereal, rice, or pasta. Limit white flour. |
| Vegetables<br>5 cups at least | Mix of dark green, yellow, or orange vegetables, beans or peas, and starchy vegetables. Consider adding more vegetables and subtracting grains. |
| Fruit<br>2½ cups | Mix the variety, but limit fruit juices. |
| Nonfat dairy products<br>3 cups | Use nonfat milk, nonfat yogurt, and nonfat cheese. |
| Meat<br>5 ounces | Choose more fish and lean poultry. Substitute beans, nuts, seeds, or tofu. |
| Fat, sugar, sodium<br>Sharply reduce | Eliminate butter, cocoa butter, cream, ice cream, and cheese. Use olive oil. Eliminate salt and refined sugar. |

At first, planning a daily menu takes some effort until new habits are well established. The following idealized example follows the Dietary Guidelines for Americans for a 1,600-calorie diet with reduced saturated fat intake, but with adequate monounsaturated fat, and omega-3 and omega-6 fatty acids.

The menu also includes abundant high-fiber, multigrain items, and is sodium restricted.

*Breakfast*
Steel cut oatmeal
Nonfat milk, 8 oz
Orange whole

*Lunch*
Black bean soup
Dark rye bread, 1 slice
Green salad with nonfat cottage cheese, lemon vinaigrette
Carrot and celery sticks
Thompson seedless grapes

*Dinner*
Poached salmon with lentil and brown rice pilaf
Steamed broccoli
Tomato salad with cucumbers and bell pepper, oil and vinegar dressing
Blackberries, 1 cup
Nonfat frozen yogurt, 8 oz

Calories 1,600, total fat 42 grams (25 percent of calories), saturated fat 5 grams, monounsaturated fat 29 grams, polyunsaturated fat 6.3 grams, fiber 40 grams, sodium 1000 milligrams

In the menu above, we assume portion size consistent with the recommendations of the U.S. Department of Agriculture diet pyramid and the portion exchanges of the diets of the American Diabetes Association. The menu includes items that are easy to measure or are low enough in calories that precision is less important. For example, oatmeal packages indicate the portion size and number of calories in a serving, and commercial bread wrappers contain similar food value information for each slice. Accuracy in measuring the small number of calories in a specific orange or serving of steamed broccoli makes little difference in calculating the day's total intake.

However, many people find portion sizes to be confusing for recipes that include multiple ingredients. How do we count portion exchanges for minestrone, jambalaya, or Mediterranean fish stew? Should we assume one portion of soup to be a cup or a bowl? Eight ounces of curried spinach soup contains one hundred calories, while cowboy soup has three hundred calories for the same eight ounces. Portion exchanges and volume measurements are sometimes confusing.

**Count calories instead of portions to personalize your menu.** Most people who are trying to lose weight rely on numbers of calories rather than using portion exchanges to give greater accuracy and flexibility. The dieter has the option of increasing or reducing the portion size to fit a personalized daily menu. Multi-ingredient recipes like minestrone, jambalaya, and Mediterranean fish stew are usually one-dish meals in our house, so each portion might be more than one serving, and we might serve a smaller portion at lunch than at dinner. For our soup recipes, we have indicated the serving size in both ounces and calories so that you can estimate the calorie difference between soups with higher or lower calories, and between a small cup and a large bowl. Likewise, beans, vegetables, pasta, couscous, or risotto might be main courses or side dishes. For fish and chicken recipes, we've assumed six-ounce portions, because markets commonly sell chicken breasts and fish fillets in those sizes. Our athletic neighbors always assume four-ounce portions of chicken or fish, because vegetables and rice or pasta are the center of their diet. They estimate smaller portions for their fish or chicken and larger for their vegetables or pasta.

The Dietary Guidelines for Americans and the U.S. Department of Agriculture diet pyramid omit alcohol, because the questionable nutritional value in alcoholic beverages does not justify the potentially harmful effects. In the next section, we discuss the hazards of alcohol and point out better alternative sources of any healthful nutrients that alcoholic beverages may contain.

# *Alcohol Can Kill in More Ways than One.*

*Key Points*

- *Many fatal accidents are alcohol-related.*
- *Accidents kill more people than does diabetes.*
- *Alcohol exacerbates several metabolic diseases.*

For many people, consumption of moderate amounts of alcohol has no apparent adverse effect. Some proponents of red wine even assert that life spans may be longer for moderate drinkers than for the population in general (Wu 2001, 3–17). However, the notion that consumption of red wine causes increased longevity is only speculation. Most cardiologists assert that "alcohol should never be recommended to patients to reduce cardiovascular risk as a substitute for the well-proven alternatives of appropriate diet, exercise, and drugs" (Vogel 2002, 7–13). In a study from Denmark, researchers showed that alcohol was associated with a slight increase in HDL-cholesterol, but the study did not confirm a cause and effect relationship, and the researchers concluded that the slight improvement noted "might be rather explained by other life-style confounders. . ." (Hansen 2005, 449–55). Among long-lived people in cultures associated with the consumption of red wine, health-promoting habits like maintenance of a normal weight, low-saturated fat intake, and more exercise may better explain their longevity, as with the population on Crete and the Mediterranean diet (Hu 2003, 2595–2596). In other long-lived populations, such as on Okinawa, consumption of alcohol is zero.

**The French paradox.** Some wine advocates point to the French paradox as evidence of a health-promoting benefit of red wine, arguing that life expectancy is longer in France than in the United States because of presumed greater red wine consumption. However, the World Health Organization (WHO) publishes comparative life expectancy data that do not support the existence of a French paradox.

**Life Expectancy, France and the United States, 1981 and 2002[9]**

| *Year* | *American Men* | *French Men* | *American Women* | *French Women* |
|---|---|---|---|---|
| 1981 | 70.4 | 70.9 | 77.6 | 78.9 |
| 2002 | 74.6 | 75.9 | 79.8 | 83.5 |

("Bulletin of the World Health Organization" 2007, 474–481 and www.who.int/whr/2003/en/facts_and_figures-en.pdf.)

A higher prevalence of obesity in the United States probably accounts for the small longevity advantage in France. For the year 2002, the World Health Organization reports that 37.8 percent of American women were obese contrasted with only 6.1 percent of French women. Among American men, 36.5 percent were obese contrasted with 7.8 percent of French men. As the obesity epidemic in the United States is relatively recent, we might expect the gap in life expectancy to widen in the coming years. Red wine consumption probably has little or no effect on longevity differences compared to the major effect of high obesity levels in the United States. (www.who.int/infobase/compare.aspx?dm=5&countries=250%2c840&year=2002&sfl=cd.0701&sex=all&agegroup=15-100).

**Antioxidants in red wine.** Red wine advocates, including some physicians, cite the theoretical benefit of antioxidants, such as resveratrol in red wine, which many speculate will retard the development of atherosclerosis, cancer, and many other degenerative diseases (Wu 2001, 3–17). Grapes and grape juice contain just as much resveratrol as red wine, as do many other fruits and nuts, including raspberries, blueberries, plums, peanuts, etc. However, fresh fruits and nuts don't seem to generate the same passionate promotion as wine. It is important to note that the quantity of antioxidants in wine, or in any other nutrient, may be far below the amount required for any theoretical biological effect on longevity (Saiko 2008, 68–94). The next section on nutritional supplements explains the current status of resveratrol

9 The most striking contrast in life expectancy was between French men (75.9 years) and French women (83.5 years) in the year 2002, a difference of 7.6 years longer life for women than for men. One possible reason is the higher prevalence of smoking among French men (40 percent) than among French women (27 percent) during the 1990s. Since most adverse effects of smoking take years to develop, life expectancy data for 2002 would reflect smoking habits in earlier decades, such as during the 1990s (www.who.int/infobase/reportviewer.aspx?rptcode=ALL&uncode=250&dm=8&surveycode=101287a15).

in a concentrated, higher-dose pill form.

**Alcohol causes accidents.** The boundary between moderate and excessive amounts of alcohol eludes many people, at least some of the time. Guidelines that various state departments of motor vehicles publish assume beverage sizes smaller than those served in most restaurants. A *Wall Street Journal* survey showed that restaurants often serve six or seven ounces of wine per glass instead of the five ounces indicated in state brochures, and a glass of draught beer in a restaurant often contains sixteen or twenty ounces, not the standard twelve. Many states allow motor vehicle drivers a maximum blood alcohol level of 0.08 percent, even though studies have shown impaired reflexes and dexterity at lower levels. Driving a motor vehicle after consuming alcohol raises an even greater danger for the elderly, because as we age, we become confused more readily from alcohol and metabolize it more slowly. Many drugs interact with alcohol to intensify the risk of driving a motor vehicle, including over-the-counter drugs like antihistamines. Complacency reigns as anyone can observe among the drivers exiting the parking lots of restaurants and bars.

During the year 2005, accidents killed 114,876 Americans and injured an estimated two and one half million. Accidents were the fifth most common cause of death in the United States, and the number-one cause in people who died before the age of fifty-five, according to the National Vital Statistics Reports of 2007. More than forty-two thousand of those accidental deaths were a result of motor vehicle crashes, and in at least 40 percent of the cases, alcohol was a factor according to the National Highway and Transportation Safety Administration (NHTSA) (http://www.nhtsa.dot.gov/people/injury/research/AlcoholCountries/other_research.htm).

The NHTSA underreports alcohol involvement in fatal crashes, because "no state reports blood alcohol concentrations for all the drivers and nonoccupants involved in fatal crashes. The missing data ranges from a few percent in some states to nearly complete absence of testing in others" (http://www-nrd.nhtsa.dot.gov/pdf/nrd-30/NCSA/Rpts/2002/00AlcoholRpt/ Alc00Chap1.htm#_VPID_2). Consequently, the actual number of alcohol-related fatal crashes in the United States greatly exceeds the 40 percent that the Fatality Analysis Reporting System reports to the NHTSA. Nevertheless, driving while under the influence of alcohol has become almost a social norm. In California, a conviction results only in a six-month loss of license.

In contrast, no amount of alcohol in the blood is tolerated in some other countries, like Sweden, where penalties are severe; consequently, the rate of accident-related deaths is much lower according to the NHTSA. Only 3.3 percent of motor-vehicle accident fatalities are alcohol-related in Sweden, contrasted with the more than 40 percent of highway accidents reported as alcohol-related in the United States (NHTSA 2002, http://www-nrd.nhtsa.dot.gov/pdf/nrd-

30/NCSA/Rpts/2002/00AlcoholRpt/Alc00Chap2.htm#_FIGURE1). If the United States were to adopt Sweden's more restrictive laws prohibiting all alcohol consumption before driving a motor vehicle, the extrapolated number of saved lives would be more than fifteen thousand per year.

**The metabolic consequences of alcohol.** In addition to accidents, alcohol can cause or aggravate numerous metabolic or degenerative diseases. Alcohol may raise blood pressure, and in the large number of people with elevated VLDL, consumption of alcohol further increases the serum triglyceride and lowers HDL, a combination known to increase the risk of heart attacks and strokes (Brunzell 2007, 1009–1017). Persons who regularly consume alcohol should be certain that they do not have a low HDL or high triglyceride problem. If in doubt, ask your physician. Alcohol consumption is also a risk factor for osteoporosis, so that persons at risk, such as those taking medications like prednisone, or anyone who has a strong family history of fractures, should abstain. Elderly people who consume alcohol are more at risk for falls, especially during the night. Of course, anyone with neurological impairment, liver disease, or any of the chronic degenerative diseases associated with alcohol should completely abstain.

In this age of greater longevity, multiple disabilities, polypharmacy, and fast automobiles, our culture has created a cocktail for an annual inflation in the rate of alcohol-related deaths.

# *Some Nutritional Supplements Promote Good Health. Some don't.*

*Key Points*

- *Vitamin B12 deficiency is common past age seventy.*
- *Folic acid deficiency causes serious birth defects.*
- *Omega-3 and omega 6 fatty acids may reduce coronary heart disease.*
- *Antioxidant supplements like vitamin E and resveratrol have doubtful benefits.*

## A. Beneficial nutritional supplements

**Vitamin B12.** Vitamin B12 deficiency is a commonly overlooked disease of the elderly that can cause anemia and serious neurological impairment, such as gait instability and memory loss. More than 30 percent of adults past the age of seventy have vitamin B12 deficiency because of a decline in production of stomach acid, called gastric achlorhydria. Dietary vitamin B12 binds to protein in food, but stomach acid breaks the bond allowing assimilation of the free vitamin B12. Since vitamin B12 in tablets is already in the free form, and not bound to protein, normal assimilation occurs even in the absence of stomach acid. The Dietary Guidelines for Americans recommend that all adults over the age of fifty take vitamin B12 supplements. As little as the five micrograms per day found in multivitamins is probably sufficient, but the higher doses in most vitamin B12 tablets is better. Readers should not confuse vitamin B12 deficiency as a result of a lack of stomach acid in the elderly with pernicious anemia, a more rare disease caused by a deficiency of a substance called intrinsic factor, which is necessary for the absorption of vitamin B12.

**Folic acid.** Folic acid deficiency, common in young women, can lead to serious neurological defects in newborn children. Taking folic acid tablets for several months before and during a pregnancy can prevent major birth defects. A recent study from Canada showed a 50 percent reduction in the number of neurological defects in newborns of mothers who had taken folic acid supplements, compared to a similar population prior to Canada's folic acid fortification program (De Wals 2007, 135).

A number of promising studies have looked at the use of folic acid supplements to prevent Alzheimer's disease, but the evidence so far has not shown any benefit (Grimley 2003, CD004514). In spite of research efforts, the causes of dementia remain mostly unknown, and so recommendations for prevention remain speculative and unsupported by experimental evidence. Older adults who choose to take folic acid should also take vitamin B12, because taking folic acid alone in the presence of mild vitamin B12 deficiency can precipitate the peripheral nerve degeneration and other neurological abnormalities associated with severe B12 deficiency.

**Iron, Calcium, and Vitamin D.** Iron and calcium tablets can interact to interfere with absorption of each other; don't take them at the same time. Young women should consider taking iron supplements, because of a high incidence of iron-deficiency anemia. Taking calcium tablets like Tums helps to prevent early development of osteoporosis, a disease more common in women and in anyone taking corticosteroids like prednisone. For adults who have little or no sun exposure, the National Osteoporosis Foundation recommends Vitamin $D_3$ supplements of 1,000 IU per day, which is approximately the same amount that humans produce during one minute of midday sun exposure.

**Fish oil, Omega-3, and Omega-6 fatty acids.** Fish oil supplements containing omega-3 and omega-6 fatty acids are now the fifth-best selling dietary supplement behind multivitamins, calcium, and vitamins C and E. Although some recent studies have failed to show "a significant reduction in cardiovascular events or mortality rate with dietary or pharmacologic omega-3 fatty acid supplementation" (Hooper 2006, 752–760), other analyses present evidence that omega-3 and omega-6 fatty acids are effective (Willett 2007, S42–45).

One such randomized clinical trial involving patients with known heart disease showed that fish oil reduced their mortality rate by suppressing fatal arrhythmias, rather than by retarding the development of atherosclerosis. The dose required to demonstrate a measurable benefit was less than one gram per day. However, at doses greater than three grams per day, fish oil also appeared to reduce blood triglyceride levels, lower blood pressure, and reduce clot formation.

On the basis of several randomized clinical trials, the American Heart Association now recommends twice a week consumption of oily fish, like salmon or mackerel, and that people with heart disease additionally take fish oil supplements, one gram per day (Breslow 2006, 1477S–1482S). An even greater amount of fish in the diet would risk higher exposure to mercury and other heavy metal toxicity, but distillation of fish oil in nutritional supplements mitigates that risk for those who require higher doses as a dietary supplement for treatment of elevated triglyceride blood levels (Oh 2008, 310).

## B. Nutritional supplements with doubtful benefit

### Antioxidant Supplements.

**Resveratrol:** Interest in high-dose antioxidant supplements arose from experiments in mice that lived longer when given resveratrol than control mice on the same diet. Based on the differences in scale and metabolic rates, an amount equal to about one hundred and fifty times the quantity of resveratrol found in red wine would be needed to adapt to humans the dose given in the mice experiments. Sources of funding are practically nonexistent for human studies of antioxidants like resveratrol, because measurable health benefits from clinical trials involving other antioxidants have been discouraging, as in the vitamin E studies below. Furthermore, researchers know that promising metabolic effects of drugs administered to mice often show no similar benefit for humans (Demetrius 2006, 66–82). Mice and men are different, pharmacologically speaking. So far, there are no published randomized clinical trials on humans that examine the safety, effectiveness, or adequate therapeutic dose of any antioxidants, including resveratrol. Nevertheless, many people now consume over-the-counter resveratrol pills of uncertain dosage that is probably not sufficient for any measurable effect on humans (Espin 2007, 2986). The Food and Drug Administration (FDA) considers resveratrol to be an experimental "nutraceutical." Until human studies demonstrate the safety, effectiveness, and appropriate dosage of antioxidants like resveratrol, the FDA and professional medical organizations will probably remain silent about recommending their use as nutrition supplements (Cucciolla 2007, 2495).

**Vitamin E**: For many years, physicians have recommended taking vitamin E, an antioxidant touted to prevent cardiovascular disease and cancer. However, several large clinical trials completed since the year 2000 have shown doubtful benefits from vitamin E in preventing heart disease, strokes, or cancer in most people. A recent Canadian randomized clinical trial enrolled 2,545 women and 6,996 men who were fifty-five years of age or older, and who had symptoms of cardiovascular disease or diabetes. Patients were randomized to receive either four hundred International Units (IU) of vitamin E or a placebo daily. The researchers concluded: "In patients at high risk for cardiovascular events, treatment with vitamin E for a mean of 4.5 years had no apparent effect on cardiovascular outcomes" (Yusuf 2000, 154).

In the Women's Health Study, 39,876 American women who were at least fifty-five years of age were followed from 1992 to 2004. Patients were randomized to receive six hundred IU of vitamin E on alternate days or a placebo. The investigators noted that vitamin E provided no overall benefit in preventing major cardiovascular events or cancer, and did not improve cardiovascular mortality or total mortality. They concluded: "These data do not support recommending vitamin E supplementation for cardiovascular disease or cancer prevention among healthy women" (Lee 2005, 56).

**Procyanidins.** Biochemists have found blood vessel dilators in red wine, grapes, berries, and other foods. Chief among these are a group of chemicals called procyanidins, popular in Europe for many years as food supplements. Some red wine advocates speculate that procyanidins are the reason for the French paradox, ignoring the probability that differences in diet and the lower prevalence of obesity may have played a role. As with antioxidants, no clinical trials on humans exist showing any measurable benefit from vasoactive substances like the procyanidins.

**Aspirin.** Aspirin disrupts platelet aggregation and so might prevent the clots that cause heart attacks or strokes, at least theoretically. Recently, six major studies involving a total of almost one hundred thousand participants have examined the results of taking aspirin to prevent heart attacks and strokes, about half the patients receiving one hundred milligrams of aspirin per day and the other half a placebo. Calculations from the combined data of the six studies, called a meta-analysis, revealed a small reduction in nonfatal heart attacks in the aspirin group, but no difference in overall cardiovascular mortality, and no difference in the incidences of strokes (Bartolucci 2006, 746). Among the patients in the Women's Health Study, mentioned earlier, investigators noted a small reduction in nonfatal strokes among women sixty-five years of age or older. However, they observed no overall improvement in mortality from either heart disease or strokes in the women who received aspirin, compared with those who received a placebo, just as in the large meta-analysis (Ridker 2005, 1293).

It is important to note that aspirin does provide protection against a heightened risk of clot formation in the period immediately following a heart attack or stroke (Van der Worp 2007, 572–578). However, the lack of overall improvement in mortality rate in multiple large studies raises the question of whether routinely taking aspirin to prevent nonfatal heart attacks or strokes justifies the risk for people with no history of heart disease. For some, taking aspirin is not an option because of a history of gastrointestinal bleeding or because of the potential of an interaction with other medications, such as anticoagulants. Anyone considering taking low-dose aspirin to prevent cardiovascular events should first consult a physician for an explanation of the potential risks and benefits as it applies to each individual. As for the procyanidins and antioxidants like vitamin E and resveratrol, either the benefit is so small as to not yet be measurable, or it doesn't exist.

# *Exercise Reduces the Risk of Coronary Heart Disease.*

*Key Points*

- *Exercise reduces the incidence of heart disease.*
- *Vigorous daily exercise works better than mild exercise.*

The new edition of the Dietary Guidelines for Americans was the first to include a strong recommendation for exercise that specifically emphasized vigorous exercise over milder activities. A reason for the change was the publication of several large, long-term studies examining the relationship between exercise and coronary heart disease, all showing a substantial risk reduction in middle-aged and older people who exercised regularly.

A study from Osaka, Japan, enrolled 76,832 men and women aged forty to seventy-nine between 1988 and 1990, and then followed them through 2003. Participants who reported exercising more than five hours per week experienced a 50 percent lower mortality rate from coronary heart disease than participants who exercised only an hour or two per week. Smokers had a higher mortality rate than nonsmokers, and exercise did not yield any improvement in that higher mortality. The authors concluded that longer hours spent exercising reduces the incidence of fatal heart attacks more than minimum hours exercising, and that exercise does not reduce the incidence of fatal coronary heart disease in smokers (Noda 2008, 471–475).

The Harvard Alumni Health Study followed 12,516 men aged thirty-nine to eighty-eight from 1977 through 1993. The amount of their exertion was logged in kilojoules per week assessing multiple activities, such as numbers of blocks walked, flights climbed, and participation in sports or recreational activities. Researchers counted the number of coronary events, including myocardial infarctions (heart attacks), onset of angina pectoris (chest pain), and numbers of deaths from coronary heart disease. Once again, the intensity of physical activities and the number of hours spent exercising per week correlated strongly with a reduction of coronary disease events (Sesso 2000, 975–980).

Another Harvard study, the Health Professionals' follow-up study, enrolled 44,452 men and followed them from 1986 to the beginning of 1998 using measurements called metabolic equivalent tasks (METs). Investigators measured physical exertion from running, weight training, and rowing. Higher intensity and longer duration of exercising was related to a reduction in new cases of coronary heart disease. Men who ran regularly experienced a 42 percent reduction in the onset of coronary heart disease compared with men who did not run. Weight training and rowing both reduced risk, but to a lesser degree than with running. Higher exercise intensity correlated with greater risk reduction (Tanasescu 2003, 1994).

Unfortunately, in none of the above studies were the subjects randomized, so that participants who exercised more may have been the same ones with other health-promoting habits. However, the stunning reduction in mortality rates from heart disease, the concurrence of the results of all three studies, the large number of participants enrolled, and the long period of follow-up justified including the recommendation for vigorous exercise in the more recent edition of the Dietary Guidelines for Americans. The Dietary Guidelines Advisory Committee could not overlook the sharp reduction in the incidence of coronary heart disease and fewer deaths from fatal myocardial infarction among the more physically active participants in the studies. Anyone who has been following the nutritional guidelines should consider adding a regular exercise regimen to further aid in weight control and to minimize the risk of disability or early death from cardiovascular disease.

**Let your pulse be your guide.** To be considered vigorous, the exercise should result in a heart rate that accelerates part of the time to within ten to twenty beats per minute of the predicted maximum rate attainable for your age. Predicted peak rate declines with age, so that a twenty- year-old person might reach two hundred beats per minute during vigorous exercise, a heart rate not normally possible for older people. Many athletes use the general rule of 220 beats per minute minus their age. A thirty-year-old might reach 190 beats per minute and a forty-year-old 180 beats per minute. By age seventy, the maximum heart rate during vigorous exercise might reach only 150 beats per minute.

Anyone can count the heart rate by feeling the carotid pulse in the neck under the angle of the jaw immediately after stopping the activity. Most athletes count for six seconds and then multiply by ten. If you count fourteen beats in six seconds, your pulse is approximately 140 beats per minute. Avoid counting for longer than six seconds, because the heart rate decelerates rapidly after stopping the exercise. Accuracy to within ten beats per minute gives all the information you need to monitor your level of exertion. Sporting goods stores sell electronic pulse measuring devices that are more accurate, but counting your approximate heart rate with your finger provides an adequate gauge of exertion level.

The heart rate should recover to about twenty beats per minute above the pre-exercise resting baseline within one minute after ending the exercise. As with the maximum heart rate, younger people recover more quickly than do older people. Anyone who experiences chest pain, undue shortness of breath, or persistent rapid pulse after exercising should consult a physician.

**Vigorous exercise takes many forms.** Examples of vigorous exercise include running, cycling, aerobic dance, and swimming, but many other alternatives require just as much exertion. The duration should total at least five hours per week based on the studies quoted above, and it is important to attain a near maximum heart rate for at least a part of the time. Researchers note that milder exercise for less time is preferable to none, but not as good as vigorous exercise for at least five hours per week (Tanasescu 2003, 1994). Some tips for success include:

- Exercise with a partner to keep each other motivated.
- Schedule a regular time each day so that it becomes a habit.
- Don't choose a form of exercise that you hate.

Finding an appropriate exercise program presents a challenge to many people who are motivated to improve their fitness. Examples of commonly available programs include aerobic dance groups, cycling clubs, swimming masters programs, and trainer-directed exercise programs offered by commercial gyms. Some commercially available programs offer only the same fixed regimen for all participants regardless of their physical capability or recent exercise history. A sedentary person who is just beginning in a program should start with stretching exercises, warm up slowly, and limit the duration of vigorous exertion to avoid injury. After several sessions, beginners can more safely increase the duration and intensity of the physical activity.

One of my older patients said that she seeks out regular participants in a program to see if they have made any progress. If she sees other lean, tight-skinned elderly participants who are working up a sweat, she has more confidence that the program may work for her too. On the other hand, if the participants are overweight and lethargic, she looks elsewhere. Just as obesity develops from bad habits that we learn from each other, we might learn good exercise habits from each other as well.

**Limited time or resources do not preclude exercise.** The old adage of taking the stairs instead of an elevator remains valid today; and a brisk walk to work or to the store serves two purposes and doesn't harm the environment. All exercise counts, but brisk climbing, walking, and running count more than just strolling. Running after work with the dog or a baby jog stroller requires only a pair of running shoes. An exercise bicycle or treadmill at home can also serve double duty if it comes equipped with a book rack. Alternatively, use headphones and listen to books on CD. You might consider measuring your pulse and keeping a log of the time spent exercising to measure your progress.

**A physical therapist can help with special needs.** Injuries can impede the ability to exercise but shouldn't become a barrier. However, trying to run through the pain risks aggravating an injury. A physical therapist can prescribe a program that won't exacerbate your injury, but will still allow you to reach reasonable exercise goals. A therapist's primary objective is to help you avoid further injury, because a second injury to the same area can greatly prolong recovery. Some public swimming pools have special exercise programs designed for injured, elderly, or disabled persons.

**Stretching:** Stretching for at least ten minutes before vigorous exercise helps to avoid muscle strains, not just for serious athletes, but more importantly, for recreational athletes. Coaches and trainers recommend stretching programs designed for specific sports, but for most recreational athletes, a general stretching routine will protect you from the muscle strains and tears that you are trying to avoid. I use practically the same stretching routine for running, swimming, and cycling. Hold each stretch until you feel tension, but not pain, and then maintain the stretch for fifteen to thirty seconds. Repeat each stretching exercise four or five times. Never bounce, as you can tear cold muscles. When you've finished stretching, begin the main exercise gradually.

Shoulder Stretch
Raise both arms over your head crossing your wrists and interlocking your fingers. Stretch as high as you can with your upper arms touching your ears.

Upper Arm Stretch
Raise one arm over your head, but bend at the elbow and touch your opposite shoulder blade. With your other hand, push back gradually on your elbow until you feel the tension.

Leg Stretch
Sit astride a bench stretching out one leg on the bench. While sitting up straight, push up with your hands to raise your body slightly until you feel tension on the back of your outstretched leg. You can then increase the tension on your leg by leaning forward slightly toward your extended foot.

Thigh Stretch
Stand holding onto a railing or chair with one hand for balance, and with the other hand grab your ankle and raise it behind your back. With your back straight, lift your ankle toward your buttocks until you feel tension in the thigh.

**Running Program.** Running requires the least amount of equipment and facilities, and so it continues to be the most popular form of vigorous exercise. Shoes wear out, however, and so you should buy new running shoes about every five hundred miles because they lose their shock absorbing capacity. Worn out shoes can lead to knee and hip injuries. Running on uneven or slanted surfaces can cause injuries, too, so seek a flat, level surface, preferably with some resilience as found on some college or high school tracks.

For beginning runners, start with brisk walking and then try jogging short distances slowly. After several weeks, begin increasing the distance, but not any faster than by five hundred meters per week. After becoming comfortable at a greater distance, begin alternating easy and challenging segments. Most well-conditioned runners can run one mile in less than ten minutes. Serious athletes run one mile in less than seven minutes.

Beginner workout, 25 minutes
- Brisk 5-minute walk
- Alternate walking and jogging for one minute each and continue for 20 minutes

Intermediate workout, 40 minutes
- Brisk 5-minute walk
- Jog for 10 minutes
- Run at moderate speed for 10 minutes
- Jog for 10 minutes
- Cool down walk for 5 minutes

Advanced workout, 60 minutes
- Brisk 5-minute walk
- Jog for 10 minutes

Run at moderate speed for 20 minutes
Jog for 10 minutes
Run at a fast pace for 10 minutes
Cool down walk for 5 minutes

**Swimming workout.** Swimming can provide vigorous exercise with minimum risk of injury and efficient use of limited time. Most communities have pools, either through organizations like the YMCA or at high schools and community colleges. Advanced swimmers may want to compete in swimming masters programs, but recreational swimmers may also enroll to improve their strokes and participate in the training workouts without having to compete in swim meets. A typical daily exercise program includes all strokes for competitive swimmers, but more senior swimmers may want to omit butterfly to avoid shoulder injuries. Below is an example of a swimming masters workout modified for recreational swimmers.

One hour, 2,200 meters

Warm Up
500 meters easy
100 kick
200 freestyle
200 back stroke
Drill
150 meters moderate—repeat 3 times for back stroke, breast stroke, and freestyle
50 kick
50 drill (see below)
50 swim
Main Set
500 meters repeated twice—5 seconds rest between each leg; 30 seconds rest between first and second round, 1 or 2 minutes rest after second round
200 freestyle, cruise (see below)
150 backstroke or breast stroke at cruise plus 15 seconds
100 freestyle, sprint
50 easy, choice of stroke
100 meters freestyle sprint for best time

Warm Down
150 meters freestyle or backstroke easy

Cruise means your usual time per 100 meters swimming a long distance. Each swimmer can measure his/her own cruise time by timing for 500 meters and dividing it by 5. Best time means sprint time for 100 meters, typically about 20 seconds faster than the cruise time. Both cruise time and best time should improve with regular workouts.

Drills help to improve your form. Examples for freestyle are:

To improve body rotation
Six kick: For each stroke, kick six times on each side
One arm: Swim each lap on the side using one arm only. Keeping the opposite arm at your side is more challenging.

To coordinate arm turnover and breathing
Catch up: Maintain one arm stretched out ahead until your hand on the recovering arm catches up and almost touches your outstretched hand.

To improve bent arm recovery
Fingertip drag: Swim dragging your fingertips in the water to encourage bending your elbow.

To improve bilateral breathing
Breathe every third stroke for a lap, then every fifth stroke for a lap, and then every seventh stroke, and repeat.

**Cycling Program.** Cycling has been enjoying increased popularity in the United States, perhaps related to the recent success of American cyclists in international professional bicycle competitions. Two fundamental requirements are a reliable bicycle and safe roads for a workout. In some of the roads around the Stanford University campus and in the Santa Cruz Mountains, cyclists almost outnumber motorists, especially on the weekends. Cycling has even been replacing golf as the "in" form of recreation for Silicon Valley executives. Two executives overheard recently asked each other: "Why don't we go play golf?" That's what the stereotypic executive does, but in Silicon Valley, "golf" is also a code word for cycling.

Riding on a level road often does not yield enough of a cardiovascular challenge to accelerate heart rate to the predicted peak. Consequently, a serious workout usually requires some hills. Racers may experience near peak cardiac acceleration on a flat segment of le Tour de France, especially during the sprint to the finish line, but recreational riders like me have a tendency to maintain only a moderate speed on a flat road.

On the day before the start of the Tour of California, I was riding on a flat road not far from the course for the next day's prologue. A peloton of professional riders on a training workout came up behind me and practically blew me off the road, stamping an exclamation point on my amateur status. On the other hand, hill climbing demands serious exertion even from easy riders.

My typical daily bicycle workout rotation varies from 1 ½ to 2 ½ hours:

Day One, 15 miles, 600 feet of elevation gain
5 miles flat terrain
2 ½ miles of climbing
2 ½ miles downhill
5 miles flat terrain

Day Two, 20 miles, 1,200 feet of elevation gain
6 miles flat terrain
4 miles of climbing
4 miles downhill
6 miles flat terrain

Day Three, 10 miles, 0 elevation gain
5 miles flat terrain
Lunch
5 miles flat terrain

All exercise programs require custom tailoring to the individual, but since exercise comes in infinite varieties, everyone can find something that works. My ninety-seven-year-old uncle finds his daily wood-chopping to be satisfying. Alternating activities, or cross training, can enhance physical fitness and improve performance for both sports. Tri-athletes juggle three activities. Two keys are avoiding injury and scheduling a regular pleasurable activity with friends. I found that among my patients who exercised regularly, there were more smiles and more bounce in their step.

# *Summary*

We can all choose to maintain an ideal weight, select healthful foods, and reduce our risk of the most common causes of disability and death. While serious illnesses can strike anyone, people who try to avoid preventable illnesses by practicing good health habits tend to be thinner and happier, and to live longer and have a reduced risk of spending many years in a nursing home. Good health habits lead to more intellectually and physically active later years. The most important principles are:

- Being consistent to attain measurable results.
- Limiting calories to avoid diabetes, high blood pressure, and atherosclerosis.
- Replacing saturated fats with olive oil, nuts, beans, and fish to improve cholesterol blood levels.
- Emphasizing fruits and vegetables that add fiber, lower blood pressure, and displace unneeded fat in the diet.
- Replacing sugar with whole grains to help control appetite and reduce the incidence of some gastrointestinal diseases.
- Restricting sodium to three thousand milligrams per day to help control blood pressure and reduce the risk of low serum potassium levels in people taking diuretics.
- Limiting or eliminating alcohol to prevent accidents, avert drug interactions, and avoid exacerbation of certain metabolic diseases.
- Participating in vigorous daily exercise to reduce the risk of cardiovascular disease.

Adhering to health-promoting principles does not require abandoning good food. The recipes that follow are mostly classic Mediterranean, Southwestern, and Asian dishes modified to fit the recommendations of the Dietary Guidelines for Americans. They emphasize fruits, vegetables, and whole grain, high-fiber ingredients, and show that enjoying culinary excellence doesn't require compromising your health. Guests at our house are usually not aware that they are consuming low-calorie, low-saturated fat meals. With a little practice, any cook can learn to substitute healthful ingredients in the recipes from any standard cookbook. It could even become a habit.

Living and even working to the age one hundred is common now. Hallmark has been printing birthday cards for centenarians. The chances of receiving such a card improve for those who practice good health habits, including a healthful diet.

Bon appétit!

# PART II
# The Recipes

The recipes that follow reflect a style found in San Francisco restaurants that emphasize fresh produce and seafood. We have modified all of the ingredients to adapt them to the Dietary Guidelines for Americans, so all entries are low in calories and contain minimal amounts of saturated fat. Most of the recipes are high in fiber and unsaturated fat. Cowboy Soup is the only recipe that includes red meat, but we boil the beef in the soup, then chill it, and completely remove all fat. We have simplified the list of ingredients and instructions to allow for ease of preparation and have tried to present them in a format convenient for a busy cook. Sue has listed below some key tricks of the trade that she has learned through the years from experience and from attending cooking schools in France.

# *Tips and Tricks*

**Bean and pasta portion size:** A one-pound package of dried beans contains twelve to thirteen servings and equals 2 ½ cups dry and 6 cups when cooked or ½ cup per serving. Each serving contains about 120 calories. One pound of dried whole-wheat spaghetti contains about nine servings of 190 calories each.

**Bouquet garni:** Tie together 4 sprigs of parsley stems, 3 sprigs fresh thyme, and 1 bay leaf to use for making stock to flavor soups, stews, and bean dishes. If you only have dried herbs, wrap and tie them in rinsed cheesecloth so you can retrieve them later.

**Capers:** Measure capers into a tea strainer and run them under cold water to remove excess salt. Capers contain plenty of salt without adding the preservative liquid, too.

**Cayenne:** Spices and herbs add complexity to many dishes, but avoid adding too much cayenne, because the intensity increases with cooking. You can always add hot sauce, salsa, or more cayenne later.

**Fish freshness:** Always smell raw fish or chicken to assure that it is fresh. Discard it if there is even a hint of an ammonia odor—better yet, don't buy it in the first place. No amount of spices or sauces can hide spoiled fish or chicken.

**Homemade croutons:** Cut leftover whole grain bread into bite-sized squares of about ½ to ¾ inches in size and shake them in a plastic bag with a small amount of olive oil and freshly ground pepper. Toast the bread chunks on a cookie sheet in an oven at 325° F for 20 minutes.

**Homemade bread crumbs:** Follow the instructions for croutons and then allow them to cool. Grind in a food processor to the desired fineness.

**Jalapeño peppers:** Use rubber gloves to protect your hands when working with hot peppers. Our daughter experienced a sleepless night because of burning hands after preparing a Mexican dinner for friends.

**Marinating chicken:** Marinating chicken before broiling flavors and tenderizes the meat. For marinades, use olive oil and mix in vinegar, lemon juice, yogurt, or buttermilk, along with spices or herbs. Place the chicken in a plastic bag with the marinade, and then put the bag of chicken in the refrigerator for at least thirty minutes.

**Nonfat chicken sausage:** If you can't find nonfat chicken or turkey sausage, grind your own in a food processor:

1 pound of ground chicken or turkey breast
1 teaspoon of ginger
1 teaspoon of powdered sage or poultry seasoning
¼ teaspoon of hot pepper flakes

**Olive oil:** Sue automatically cuts in half the amount of olive oil in published recipes. Most of our guests can't tell the difference, and since olive oil contains 124 calories per tablespoon, the reduction in calories can be substantial. Consider using citrus-flavored olive oils to add interest to steamed fresh vegetables. Many specialty markets carry a variety of flavored olive oils, but you can also order them online (www.Pasolivo.com).

**Peeling potatoes:** Sue doesn't bother to peel the potatoes for most of our soups and stews, especially when she uses red-skinned, yellow Finn, Yukon gold, or new potatoes, but she does peel them for mashed potatoes or Dutch mash. She prefers Idaho or Maine potatoes for baking.

**Peeling red bell peppers:** Cut the red bell peppers in quarters, and then place them under the broiler for about ten or twelve minutes to blacken and blister. Cover them with aluminum foil to trap the steam while they cool, and then you can easily peel off the skin before slicing them.

**Poaching or steaming fish:** Many French chefs recommend against adding lemon juice, wine, or vinegar to the poaching liquid because the fish becomes soft and macerated. Use plain water and add a few herbs if you like.

**Powdered nonfat milk:** Add a ½ cup of nonfat milk powder to 2 cups of nonfat milk for cooking. It increases the body for very little extra calories. Use powdered milk for bread recipes that require milk to avoid the extra step of scalding the milk. Powdered milk is already scalded.

**Roasting nuts:** For garnishing dishes with nuts, roast them at 320° F for twenty minutes to bring out the aroma.

**Roasting vegetables:** Tossing chopped vegetables in a plastic bag with a little olive oil and then roasting them in an oven for thirty minutes at 375° F brings out a nutty flavor and adds depth to many dishes. This works especially well for most root vegetables, summer and winter squash, eggplant, and bell peppers.

**Scorched pans:** Sprinkle onto the scorched area a generous amount of an abrasive cleaner and add 1 or 2 cups of hot water to make a slurry. Allow it to sit for two hours. You can then easily peel off the scorched layer. The pan will emerge unharmed.

**Sticking pans or rice cookers:** At the end of cooking, turn off the heat and cover, allowing the dish to sit for two or three minutes. Rice, couscous, or other foods will not stick to the pan and the cleanup will be easier.

**Sweating onions:** Sweating onions means to fry slowly in a small amount of oil at a low to medium temperature, usually for about ten to fifteen minutes. The onions become translucent and slightly caramelized instead of brown, a preferable result for most Mediterranean dishes. When a recipe calls for sweating the onions and garlic together, add the garlic near the end to avoid burning, because burned garlic gives off an unpleasant sulfur-like taste.

**Tender chicken:** After broiling chicken breasts, cover them with a lid or with aluminum foil for about ten minutes before slicing. The inside will continue to cook, but you will avoid the rubber-chicken toughness associated with institutional food. Try to limit broiling to seven minutes on each side.

**Yogurt garnish:** Instead of sour cream, the addition of a dollop of nonfat Greek or Russian yogurt to a bean or whole grain dish completes the mixture of amino acids to make complete protein.

**Zest**: Several of the recipes call for strips of citrus rind, approximately 1 to 1 ½ inches in length. A special zesting tool is inexpensive and essential for efficiency and better results. Always do the zesting before slicing the lemon or orange. Trying to zest one half of a lemon or orange is clumsy and frustrating.

# *Kitchen Tools*

Efficient preparation requires a well-equipped kitchen that has just the right tools. Some cooks collect too many unused kitchen utensils that clutter and obstruct efficient operation. We have found the following list to be indispensable. Every tool has its place to avoid the annoyance of having to search for the right implement, and Sue ruthlessly banishes any interlopers that find their way to a reserved space. Every New Year's Day, she clandestinely removes to the barn all of those well-meaning culinary Christmas presents that dare to languish unused in our kitchen cabinets.

**Power tools**
Food processor
Mixer with bread hook
Handheld blender
Rice cooker

**Pots and Pans** (We use French copper pots with stainless steel linings. Our 12-inch skillet is heavy cast iron.)
8-inch non-stick skillet
10-inch skillet with lid
12-inch heavy cast-iron skillet
Two 3½-quart covered sauce pots
5-quart covered Dutch oven
8-quart covered pasta pot
Broiling pan
Cookie sheets
Roasting pan
Angel food cake pan
Pizza stone

**Knives**
3 ½-inch paring knife
6-inch boning knife
6-inch tomato knife
7-inch utility knife
9-inch chef's knife
9-inch bread knife
Knife sharpener

**Special Aids**
Small glass citrus squeezer
Tea strainer
Salad spinner
Colander
Measuring cups and spoons
Gravy separator
Two cutting boards

**Hand Tools**
Long-handled stirring spoon
Slotted spoon
Ladle
Vegetable peeler
Tongs
Spatulas
Whisks
Scissors
Zester or microplane grater
Tweezers for removing fish bones

# *Soup*

## Stocks for Soups and Sauces

Commercial sources for stock bases save time, and the high quality of many brands make them a convenient ingredient. However, many cooks prefer to make their own stocks for a fresher taste and reduced sodium content. All of the stocks below contain almost no calories and almost no sodium.

### Vegetable Stock

(makes about 5 cups)

Bouquet garni
- 4 sprigs parsley stems
- 3 sprigs fresh thyme
- 1 bay leaf

1 leek, white portion only
1 whole onion with skins left on to color the broth
2 garlic cloves
2 stalks celery
½ cup carrots
½ cup turnips
½ cup parsnips
1 tablespoon marjoram

1. Sweat ½ cup finely chopped onions in 1 tablespoon olive oil.
2. Wash the vegetables and cut them into large pieces.
3. Submerge all the ingredients in 6 cups of water, and simmer covered for 1 ½ hours.
4. Strain and discard the vegetables.
5. Refrigerate the stock, or use it immediately for homemade vegetable soup.

## Fish Stock

(makes about 3 cups)

1 to 1 ½ pounds fish bones and tails, but avoid gills. Avoid salmon and other strongly flavored fish. Use shells from shrimp or crabs.
½ cup onions
½ cup celery
¼ cup carrots
Bouquet garni (see Vegetable Stock)
4 cloves
6 white peppercorns
½ cup dry white wine or 2 tablespoons lemon juice

1. Wash and chop the vegetables into large pieces.
2. Combine all the ingredients in 3 cups of water and simmer uncovered for 15 minutes, no longer.
3. Strain and use immediately.

## Chicken Stock

Slow simmering helps develop a richer stock for stews and soups. Strain and discard the bones and vegetables, and then allow the broth to cool in order to remove any fat. Your reward will be a true flavor enhancer for your recipes. Some cooks pour homemade stock into ice cube trays and freeze it for use later with steamed vegetables as a special treat.

### White Chicken Stock

(makes about 10 cups)

4 pounds chicken carcass/bones
2 carrots
8 ounces of onions
8 ounces of leeks
8 garlic cloves, unpeeled
Bouquet garni (see Vegetable Stock)
1 quart water

1. Wash and peel the vegetables and cut them into large pieces.
2. Submerge the chicken bones and vegetables in a large covered pot of water and bring to a boil. Simmer for two hours, strain, cool, and refrigerate.
3. Lift any fat from the top. Reheat to use immediately, or keep refrigerated for up to 7 days or several months in the freezer.

**Brown Chicken Stock**
(makes about 10 cups)

4 pounds chicken carcass/bones
2 carrots
8 ounces of onions
8 ounces of leeks
8 garlic cloves, unpeeled
4 celery stalks
Bouquet garni (see Vegetable Stock)
3 tablespoons tomato purée
3 quarts water

1. Place the chicken bones in a large oven-proof pot and brown them in the oven at 400° F for 20 minutes.
2. Chop the carrots, celery, onions, garlic, and leeks into large pieces and add to the pot.
3. Return the pot to the oven for 20 minutes more. Move the pot to the stove top.
4. Then add the 3 quarts of water, bouquet garni, and the tomato concentrate. Cover and simmer for 1 to 2 hours.
5. Strain and discard all but the liquid. Refrigerate overnight and lift off any fat from the top. May keep refrigerated up to 7 days or in the freezer for several months.

## Minestrone

Mediterranean cooks use whatever vegetables are ready from their garden or market to make minestrone, and so the soup varies by the season. Sometimes the chef adds left-over pasta, but the constant ingredients are tomatoes and beans. The flavor improves overnight in the refrigerator. The soup is low in calories and saturated fat, while rich in fiber. By using homemade vegetable stock, you can reduce the sodium to only 30 milligrams per serving.

1 cup beans cooked: cannellini, Great Northern, cranberry, kidney, or chick-peas
4 cups homemade vegetable broth
½ cup onion, finely chopped
2 garlic cloves, crushed
1 tablespoon olive oil
1 large celery rib, diced
2 carrots, diced
1 potato, diced
3 small zucchini, diced
3 small yellow crookneck squash, diced
1 cup cabbage, finely-sliced
½ cup acorn or butternut squash
6 medium-sized tomatoes, diced
1 cup brown rice or whole wheat pasta, cooked
¼ teaspoon cayenne
1 teaspoon oregano
1 bay leaf

1. Soak beans overnight and boil 1 ½ hours until tender.
2. Sweat the onion, celery, and garlic in olive oil for 10 minutes in a soup pot. Add the cayenne and oregano near the end.
3. Add the beans, carrots, potatoes, acorn squash, tomatoes, bay leaf, and broth, and simmer for about 30 minutes.
4. Add the zucchini, yellow crookneck squash, and cabbage, and simmer for an additional 5 to 7 minutes.
5. Add the cooked brown rice or whole wheat pasta just before serving.

Makes 2 quarts and serves eight 8-ounce portions
180 calories per serving, 2.9 g total fat (14 percent of calories), 0.4 g saturated, 1.8 g monounsaturated, 0.6 polyunsaturated, 0 cholesterol, 30 mg sodium, 7.6 g fiber

## Winter Squash Soup with Ginger

This spicy winter potage makes an elegant first course. Alternatively, serve it together with a green salad and dark chocolate rye bread for lunch.

2 cups butternut squash peeled, cut into 1-inch cubes
2 carrots in 1-inch slices
1 redskin potato, 3-inch diameter, peeled and diced
½ onion, diced
1 clove garlic, pressed
2 inches fresh ginger, peeled and diced
1 tablespoon canola oil
1 quart chicken broth
½ teaspoon poultry seasoning
¼ cup toasted sunflower seeds
¼ cup lemon juice

1. Fry the onions and ginger on medium low in vegetable oil for 5 minutes.
2. Add the vegetables and continue to cook until they begin to brown in about 5 minutes.
3. Add the broth and the poultry seasoning and simmer for 1 hour until the vegetables are soft.
4. Purée with handheld blender and add lemon juice.
5. Serve in soup bowls. Garnish with sunflower seeds.

Makes 1½ quarts and serves six 8-ounce portions
120 calories per serving, 5.0 g total fat (35 percent of calories), 0.6 g saturated, 2.2 g monounsaturated, 1.9 g polyunsaturated, 0 cholesterol, 200 mg sodium, 4.7 g fiber

## Curried Spinach Soup

Our daughter Helen won a prize from *Better Homes and Gardens* for her recipe of spinach soup in the January 2004 issue. Sue modified her own version to comply with the recommendations of the Dietary Guidelines for Americans. Helen can't tell the difference.

1 pound fresh spinach, washed and stems trimmed
1 large potato, peeled and chopped
½ cup green onions, sliced
1 tablespoon olive oil
⅓ cup flour
2 teaspoons curry powder
4 cups chicken broth
1 tablespoon lemon juice
8 ounces nonfat yogurt

1. In a large soup pot, sauté the potato and green onion in 1 tablespoon of olive oil for about 10 minutes or until the potato is soft.
2. Add the flour and curry powder for the last 2 minutes of cooking.
3. Add the spinach, cover, and cook for no more than 2 minutes to wilt the spinach.
4. Turn up the heat and add the chicken broth slowly, stirring until thickened.
5. Purée the mix with a hand blender until smooth.
6. Warm (don't boil) the nonfat yogurt and lemon juice in a microwave and stir it into the purée. Don't boil the soup after adding the yogurt, or it will separate into curds.
7. Serve warm with croutons. (see Tips and Tricks)

Makes 1½ quarts and serves six 8-ounce portions
100 calories per serving, 2.2 g total fat (20 percent of calories), 0.1 g saturated, 1.8 g monounsaturated, 0.2 g polyunsaturated, 0 cholesterol, 300 mg sodium, 1.4 g fiber

## Split Pea Soup

I used to make split pea soup during the weekend as a medical student, and then refrigerate or freeze part of it. Reheated, it became my nightly dinner throughout a week when there wasn't time to cook. This Mediterranean version of split pea soup with oregano and garlic dresses up the basic student version. *Herbes de Provence* contain thyme, savory, marjoram, and oregano.

1 pound dried split peas
3 large carrots, finely chopped
2 small red potatoes, chopped
1 onion, chopped
2 cloves of garlic, pressed
1 tablespoon olive oil
4 cups of chicken stock and 4 cups water
1 teaspoon *herbes de Provence*
1 teaspoon black pepper

1. Sweat the onions, garlic, herbes de Provence, and black pepper in olive oil in a soup pot for about 10 minutes.
2. Add the carrots, potatoes, split peas, and chicken stock, and simmer uncovered for one hour, stirring occasionally to avoid burning in the bottom of the pot. Add water as needed.
3. Serve with a salad and hardy whole grain bread.

Makes 2 quarts and serves eight 8-ounce portions
100 calories per serving, 1.8 g total fat (16 percent of calories), 0.2 g saturated, 1.3 g monounsaturated, 0.2 g polyunsaturated, 0 cholesterol, 200 mg sodium, 6.5 g fiber

## Navy Bean Soup

This Mediterranean soup is easy to prepare and improves with refrigeration. When time is short, reheating a bowl in a microwave provides a satisfying meal. Serve it with hardy whole grain bread and a green salad.

½ pound Great Northern (Navy) beans
1 large onion, chopped
2 garlic cloves, pressed
1 tablespoon olive oil
2 twigs (4-inch) of fresh rosemary
1 quart of homemade chicken stock
1 bay leaf
¼ teaspoon black pepper

1. Soak the beans overnight.
2. Sweat the onions and garlic in olive oil for 10 minutes.
3. Add the beans, chicken stock, rosemary, black pepper, and bay leaf. Cover and simmer on low for about 1 hour.
4. Remove the rosemary twigs and bay leaf and purée the soup with a handheld electric blender, leaving chunks of beans intact for texture.

Makes 5 ½ cups and serves five 8-ounce portions
155 calories per serving, 3.2 g total fat (19 percent of calories), 0.5 g saturated, 2.0 g monounsaturated, 0.4 g polyunsaturated, 0 g cholesterol, 60 mg sodium, 6.9 g fiber

## Black Bean Soup

Many cultures claim ownership of black bean soup, but this version has a Southwestern flavor with jalapeño and cilantro. Like white bean soup, it can be refrigerated and served later. By limiting the amount of chicken stock, it becomes Mexican black beans to serve with tortillas, salsa, and brown rice. For another variation, blend in 1 cup of mashed butternut squash.

½ pound of black beans
1 red bell pepper, chopped
2 celery stalks, chopped
1 onion, chopped
1 small carrot, finely diced
1 can (14.5-ounce) diced tomatoes
2 tablespoon tomato paste
3 cups homemade chicken stock
3 garlic cloves, pressed
1 jalapeño pepper, finely chopped with seeds and membranes removed
3 twigs of fresh cilantro, chopped, or cilantro seeds
1 tablespoon olive oil
1 tablespoon cumin
1 tablespoon oregano
1 teaspoon paprika

1. Soak the beans overnight and boil for about 1 hour. Set aside.
2. Sauté the onion, garlic, celery, carrot, red bell pepper, jalapeño, and cilantro in the olive oil for about 15 minutes until all vegetables are soft.
3. Add the tomatoes, tomato paste, chicken stock, and beans and simmer for about 30 minutes.
4. Purée the soup with a handheld electric blender, leaving chunks of beans intact for texture.

Makes 1½ quarts and serves six 8-ounce portions
155 calories per serving, 2.7 g total fat (16 percent of calories), 0.4 g saturated, 1.7 g monounsaturated, 0.2 g polyunsaturated, 0 cholesterol, 150 mg sodium, 7.0 g fiber

## Cowboy Soup

Cowboys are hardy and so is this bean and beef soup, the only recipe in the book that calls for red meat. In order to keep the calories and fat content low, carefully remove the fat from the chilled broth after refrigerating overnight. The little cowboys in our house were big fans.

2 pounds beef bones (short ribs)
9 cups of cold water
½ cup of dried pinto beans soaked overnight
½ cup of black-eyed peas soaked overnight
½ teaspoon of crushed red peppers or ¼ teaspoon cayenne
1 large onion, diced
2 stalks of celery with greens, chopped
1 medium-sized potato, finely diced
1 clove of garlic, pressed
1 tablespoon olive oil
1 bay leaf

1. Boil bones in the water for 4 hours.
2. Strain liquid through a colander and chill broth overnight; lift fat from the surface.
3. Strip any visible fat from the meat and discard. Save the lean meat.
4. Simmer the beans and black-eyed peas in water until tender, 1 ½ to 2 hours, and drain.
5. Sweat the onion, garlic, and red peppers in olive oil for 10 minutes, and combine with the beans, meat, celery, broth, and bay leaf. Simmer for 1 ½ hours.
6. Add the diced potatoes for the last 20 minutes.

Makes 2 quarts and serves eight 8-ounce portions
180 calories per serving, 4.5 g total fat (22 percent of calories), 1.8 g saturated, 2.0 g monounsaturated, 0.6 g polyunsaturated, 10 mg cholesterol, 25 mg sodium, 8.0 g fiber

## Fish Chowder (Cod, Halibut, Scallops, Oysters)

San Francisco firemen invented this hardy, milk-based seafood soup that can be adapted to any white fish, oysters, or scallops, alone or in combination. Serve it with plenty of crusty whole grain bread and ring the fire gong.

1 pound of white fish in 1-inch pieces, scallops, or 1 pint of fresh oysters with liquor
½ onion, chopped
1 stalk celery, chopped
1 red bell pepper, chopped
1 large carrot, sliced
4 small or 2 medium red-skinned potatoes, diced
1 cup frozen corn
1 tablespoon canola oil
¼ cup chopped fresh parsley
½ teaspoon thyme leaves
¼ teaspoon black pepper
⅛ teaspoon cayenne
½ cup of powdered nonfat milk
4 cups of nonfat milk
2 tablespoons flour

1. Boil the carrots and potatoes until tender, about 10 minutes. Drain.
2. Sweat the onion, celery, and red bell pepper in olive oil for 10 minutes, stirring in the flour, black pepper, cayenne, and thyme during the final 1 to 2 minutes.
3. Stir the milk powder into the liquid nonfat milk with a whisk and add to the sweated vegetables. Bring to a boil stirring constantly to thicken the broth
4. Add the drained carrots, potatoes, and frozen corn and bring the heat back to boiling.
5. Add the fish. Bring back to a boil, cover, and turn off the heat.
6. Add the parsley

Makes 1½ quarts and serves six 8-ounce portions
180 calories per serving, 2.8 g total fat (10 percent of calories), 0.3 g saturated, 1.8 g monounsaturated, 0.6 g polyunsaturated, 18 mg cholesterol, 100 mg sodium, 3.2 g fiber

## Clam Chowder, Manhattan Style

New Englanders refuse to acknowledge the existence of Manhattan clam chowder; nevertheless, this tomato-based soup is delicious, and the flavor improves with storage overnight in the refrigerator. Reheat it later when large numbers of hungry guests arrive at odd hours. Our grandchildren don't come to see us; they come for Sue's cooking.

large can of shucked sea clams and juice
1 large onion, finely chopped
4 tablespoons flour
1 tablespoon olive oil
2 cups of red-skinned potatoes, diced
2 cans (14.5-ounce) of diced tomatoes
2 carrots, diced
3 cups fish stock or water
½ cup tomato paste
1 bay leaf
1 teaspoon sage or poultry seasoning
1 teaspoon black pepper
(Optional: 1 stalk celery, finely chopped)

1. Sweat the onion in olive oil for 10 minutes.
2. Stir in the flour and cook for an additional 2 minutes.
3. Add all of the rest of the ingredients along with 3 cups of fish stock or water.
4. Cover and simmer for about 30 minutes until the carrots and potatoes are soft.
5. Refrigerate overnight. Reheat and serve the next day.

Makes 3 quarts and serves twelve 8-ounce portions
190 calories per serving, 1.8 g total fat (9 percent of calories), 0.2 g saturated, 1.3 g monounsaturated, 0.2 g polyunsaturated, 120 mg cholesterol, 575 mg sodium, 1.1 g fiber

## Mediterranean Fish Stew

Mediterranean cooks prepare this tomato-based fishermen's stew from Naples to Marseilles to Barcelona, and they serve it with lots of bread to soak up the broth. It works with almost any white fish or shell fish or both. Marcel Pagnol describes a bouillabaisse like this in his trilogy of plays about Marseilles, *Marius, Fanny,* and *César*.

1 to 1½ pounds white fish: sablefish, cod, halibut, or orange roughy
(Optional: ½ lb calamari, scallops, shrimp, or other shell fish)
1 medium carrot, diced
1 red-skinned potato, diced
3 ripe tomatoes or 1 can crushed tomatoes
½ medium onion, chopped
3 garlic cloves, pressed
1½ cups fish stock, clam juice, or water
(Optional: 1 cup dry white wine instead of 1 cup of fish stock or water)
1 tablespoon olive oil
1 teaspoon minced thyme
1 piece (2-inch) of orange peel
1½ teaspoons cumin
¼ teaspoon cayenne
2 tablespoons minced parsley

1. Sweat the onions and garlic in olive oil on low, but don't brown.
2. Add the carrots, tomatoes, stock, spices, orange peel, and white wine, and simmer for 10 minutes uncovered. Then add the potatoes and simmer covered for another 30 minutes.
3. Add the seafood, bring back to boiling, cover, simmer for 2 minutes, and turn off the heat. Don't overcook the seafood.
4. Add the parsley and serve immediately.

Makes 5 cups and serves five 8-ounce portions
200 calories per serving, 4.2 g total fat (18 percent of total calories), 0.5 g saturated, 2.3 g monounsaturated, 0.7 g polyunsaturated, 30 mg cholesterol, 200 mg sodium, 1.9 g fiber

# *Seafood*

## Three Sauces for Sautéed Fish

The following recipes give variety to sautéed fish. Preparation is easy and the cooking time is short, but the results are like the best San Francisco restaurants, except that we substitute olive oil for butter. Dry the fish with a paper towel and press it into the preferred coating. Refrigerate for at least 30 minutes to set the coating. Sauté the fish in a minimal amount of olive oil for 3 to 4 minutes per side. Sauté tuna for only 1 to 2 minutes per side. Remove the fish and deglaze the pan to make the mustard or caper sauce.

1. **Crushed nuts or seeds**
   — Grind freshly roasted almonds, pistachios, macadamia nuts, peanuts, or sesame seeds in a food processor or coffee grinder. Use ½ ounce per serving.
   — Sprinkle half ground nuts or seeds onto waxed paper or a flat plate and press fish onto the coating. Sprinkle the other half on the fish. Press gently and refrigerate for at least 30 minutes.

80 calories per serving, 7.6 g total fat, (80 percent of calories), 0.6 g saturated, 4.8 g monounsaturated, 1.6 g polyunsaturated, 0 cholesterol, 8 mg sodium, 4 g fiber

2. **Capers**
   — For each serving, mix 1 tablespoon flour and ½ teaspoon Cajun seasoning.
   — Coat the fish and refrigerate for at least 30 minutes.
   — Add juice of ½ lemon and ½ tablespoon of capers per serving to the pan after the fish is sautéed.

For variation, substitute orange juice or dry white wine for the lemon juice. Also, try adding 1 tablespoon balsamic or sherry vinegar to the juice or wine. Substitute other herbs for the Cajun seasoning, including cumin, rosemary, dill, parsley, thyme, cilantro, basil, mint, or oregano.

40 calories per serving, < 0.1 g total fat, 50 mg sodium

**3. Mustard sauce**

- — Coat each fish fillet with 1 tablespoon of Dijon mustard per serving
- — Refrigerate for at least 30 minutes.
- — Sprinkle a few sesame seeds on top of the fish.
- — Use 1 tablespoon white wine per serving to deglaze the pan.

30 calories per serving, < 0.1 g total fat, 50 mg sodium

## Steamed Salmon, Rice Noodles, and Spinach

This recipe fuses Japanese-style steamed fish with a New England clam bake, which isn't a bake at all, but a mix of steamed clams and lobster. Serve the fish on top of the rice noodles and spinach. Add low-sodium soy sauce, wasabi mustard, and fresh ginger. It's ichiban Down East.

Rice noodles and spinach
¼ onion, coarsely chopped
2 ounces cellophane rice noodles
8 ounce package of washed spinach

1. Place about 1 inch of water in the bottom of a large pot along with the chopped onion, bring to a boil, and turn off the heat.
2. Add the rice noodles to the pot with the spinach on top.
3. Cover, bring to a boil and turn off.
4. Let the steamed noodles and spinach sit for at least 5 minutes. Drain in a colander.

Salmon
2 salmon filets, about 6 ounces each
1½ inches ginger root, peeled and chopped

1. Place the ginger root in 1 inch of water in a covered poaching pan and bring to a boil.
2. Turn off and let sit for about 5 minutes.
3. Add the fish, bring to a boil again, turn off, and let it sit for another 5 minutes.

**Optional sauces or garnishes**

- Rice vinegar or distilled vinegar with zest of peeled ginger root
- ¼ cup of low-sodium soy sauce with 1 teaspoon sesame oil and chopped green onions
- Pickled ginger

Serves 2
300 calories per serving, 8.8 g total fat (14 percent of calories), 1.6 g saturated, 3.5 g monounsaturated, 4.1 g polyunsaturated, 75 mg cholesterol, 76 mg sodium, 1.1 g fiber

## Poached Salmon with a Lentil and Brown Rice Pilaf

Real fishermen say that poaching is the only method for salmon, referring to the cooking of course. French chefs advise against adding lemon juice, wine, or vinegar to the poaching liquid because they soften and macerate the salmon. Serve the salmon on top of the pilaf and garnish with two sprigs of broccoli for color. Start by preparing the lentils and rice; poach the fish at the last minute.

Salmon
4 salmon filets (6 ounces each)

1. Place ½ inch of water in a sauté pan and bring to a boil.
2. Place the fish in the boiling water and bring back to a boil. Cover, turn off the heat, and allow to stand for about 5 minutes. Don't overcook the salmon.
3. Serve on top of the lentil and brown rice pilaf.

Sauce
2 tablespoons olive oil
2 Meyer lemons for juice and zest

1. Place all the ingredients together in a small sauté pan and heat on low until they become fragrant—about 3 minutes.
2. Pour over the salmon.

Serves 4
345 calories per serving, 13 g total fat (32 percent of calories), 2.0 g saturated, 6.0 g monounsaturated, 4.8 g polyunsaturated, 75 mg cholesterol, 90 mg sodium, 1 g fiber

Lentils
¼ pound dried lentils
1 cup steamed brown rice
½ onion, chopped
1 stalk celery, chopped
1 carrot, chopped
1 clove garlic, pressed
½ tablespoon olive oil
1 Meyer lemon for juice and zest
1 cup of chicken stock
¼ teaspoon black pepper
1 tablespoon mint leaves, chopped

1. Sweat the onions, garlic, and pepper in a pan for about 10 minutes.
2. Add the lentils, celery, carrot, lemon zest, and chicken stock, cover and simmer for 20 minutes.
3. Add the brown rice and stir in the lemon juice.
4. Serve as a base for the salmon with mint leaf garnish.

Serves 4
195 calories per serving, 7.3 g total fat (34 percent of calories), 1.0 g saturated, 5.2 g monounsaturated, 1.3 g polyunsaturated, 0 mg cholesterol, 60 mg sodium, 8.3 g fiber

## Oven-Poached Halibut with Spinach

The secret to baking fish is minimum time in a hot oven. This Mediterranean recipe has zest, literally, and will delight the pepper lover. Try it with cod, orange roughy, or sablefish. Serve the fish on a bed of steamed spinach.

2 pieces of halibut (6 ounces each)
1 cup fish stock or water
½ tablespoon olive oil
6 whole black peppercorns
1 Meyer lemon for juice
Zest strips from the lemon
¼ teaspoon cayenne
4 or 5 twigs of flat-leaf parsley, chopped

1. Preheat oven to 425° F and heat the fish stock, lemon zest, olive oil and peppercorns in a small roasting dish to near boiling.
2. Place the fish in the hot liquid, adding hot water if necessary so that the liquid nearly covers the fish. Sprinkle a little cayenne on the fish.
3. Roast for about 8 minutes.
4. Serve the fish on top of steamed spinach. Spoon the lemon juice and some of the poaching sauce over the fish.

Makes 2 servings
200 calories per serving, 4.4 g total fat (10 percent of calories), 0.5 g saturated, 2.4 g monounsaturated, 1.4 g polyunsaturated, 40 mg cholesterol, 90 mg sodium, 0 g fiber

## Whitefish in a Tomato Sauce

A plate of sautéed fish, tomatoes, onion, and garlic rewards the Sicilian fisherman at the end of the day. Serve it with a crusty loaf of whole grain bread or pasta and a green salad. Almost any white fish works, such as sablefish, Alaskan cod, halibut, or orange roughy.

2 fish filets (6 ounces each)
1 tablespoon flour for dusting the fish
1 tablespoon of Cajun seasoning
1 tablespoon olive oil
1 medium onion, chopped
2 garlic cloves, pressed
1 can (14.5-ounce) diced tomatoes, drained
2 tablespoons tomato paste or ketchup
1 tablespoon cumin
¼ cup minced cilantro

1. Sweat the onion, garlic, and cumin in olive oil for 10 minutes.
2. Add the tomatoes and simmer for an additional 10 minutes.
3. Stir in the minced cilantro.
4. Dust the fish with flour and Cajun seasoning in a plastic bag, and sauté in olive oil over medium heat for 3 minutes per side.
5. Pour the tomato and onion mix over the fish during the last minute and serve immediately.

Serves 2
245 calories per serving, 7.9 g total fat (29 percent of calories), 1.0 g saturated, 5.2 g monounsaturated, 0.9 g polyunsaturated, 40 mg cholesterol, 640 mg sodium, 0.7 g fiber

## Sablefish and New Potatoes with a Honey-Mustard Glaze

French chefs combine the sweetness of the honey with the richness of the sablefish. The key here is roasting the potatoes for 45 minutes first, while baking the fish in a hot oven for only 8 minutes. Serve with steamed spinach or other green vegetable.

4 sablefish fillets (about 6 ounces each)
16 to 20 small new potatoes
1 tablespoon olive oil
¼ cup Dijon mustard
2 tablespoons honey

1. Shake the potatoes and oil in a plastic bag and place them in a 10 inch x 15 inch baking pan. Roast at 425° F for about 45 minutes. Move the potatoes to one end of the pan.
2. Combine the honey and mustard and coat the potatoes with half and the fish with half.
3. Bake the potatoes and fish for an additional 8 minutes.
4. Serve the pan juices on the fish and potatoes.

Makes 4 servings
400 calories per serving, 4.7 g total fat (10 percent of calories), 0.4 g saturated, 2.7 g monounsaturated, 0.4 g polyunsaturated, 60 mg cholesterol, 275 mg sodium, 2.2 g fiber

## Tuna with Olives, Red Bell Pepper, Capers, and Sun-Dried Tomatoes

Mediterranean chefs know more variations for tuna than just *la salade Niçoise.* Cut the red peppers into quarters, and then place them under the broiler for about 10 or 12 minutes to blacken and blister the skin. Cover them with aluminum foil to trap the steam while they cool, and then you can easily peel off the skin before slicing them. Spoon the sauce on the whole-wheat spaghetti. Sear the tuna briefly and serve it on top. Steamed broccoli adds color.

2 tuna steaks (about 4 to 6 ounces each)
1 tablespoon sun-dried tomatoes, chopped
2 Roma tomatoes, chopped
2 tablespoons tomato paste or ketchup
¼ cup black olives, pitted and chopped
¼ red bell pepper, roasted, peeled, and chopped
¼ cup onion, chopped
2 tablespoons capers, rinsed
3 cloves garlic, pressed
1 tablespoon olive oil
4 sprigs parsley, chopped
Black pepper to taste

1. Broil the red bell pepper until the skin blisters, about 10 to 12 minutes; then cover with aluminum foil to capture the steam while cooling. When cool enough, peel and finely chop the pepper.
2. Sweat the onion and garlic in a small amount of olive oil for 10 minutes.
3. Stir in the chopped tomatoes, sun-dried tomatoes, tomato paste, red bell pepper, and olives. Simmer for about 20 minutes, adding the capers and parsley at the end.
4. Sauté the tuna in a small amount of olive oil for 2 minutes per side. Remove from the heat and allow to sit for 5 minutes to retain the juices.
5. Slice the tuna into ¼- to ½-inch-thick strips and serve over whole wheat spaghetti. Spoon the sauce along the top of the tuna.

Serves 2
325 calories per serving with spaghetti, 13 g total fat (36 percent of calories), 1.3 g saturated, 9 g monounsaturated, 1.1 g polyunsaturated, 63 mg cholesterol, 300 mg sodium, 2.9 g fiber

## Polynesian Grilled Tuna

Polynesian dishes work well served with fresh Hawaiian fruit and brown rice. Alternatively, serve it with spinach, steamed or in a salad. Garnish the tuna with pickled ginger. Don't overcook it.

4 tuna steaks, ahi or tombo (about 6 ounces each)
3 tablespoons lime juice
1 glove garlic, pressed
1 tablespoons sesame oil
2 tablespoons reduced-sodium soy sauce
1 tablespoons minced fresh ginger
Lime wedges

1. Place the tuna, lime juice, soy sauce, sesame oil, ginger, and garlic into a plastic bag and shake. Marinate the fish for at least 1 hour in the refrigerator. Discard marinade.
2. Grill over hot coals, about 2 minutes per side.
3. Serve with lime wedges, papaya, mango, or fresh pineapple.

Serves 4
200 calories per serving, 5.0 g total fat (22 percent of calories), 0.7 g saturated, 2.0 g monounsaturated, 1.5 g polyunsaturated, 71 mg cholesterol, 370 mg sodium, 0.1 g fiber

## Salmon or Crab Cakes

Wild Pacific salmon makes wonderful fish cakes that can be served with rice or wheat berry pilaf and the caper sauce found at the beginning of the seafood section. Garnish with a few twigs of watercress. Alternatively, substitute crab in place of the salmon for a recipe like the one at the Hayes Street Grill, the best San Francisco restaurant for crab cakes. Sometimes they offer the crab cakes as the centerpiece of a salad. Go early because they run out.

2 salmon filets (6 ounces each) or 12 ounces crabmeat
3 tablespoons egg substitute
3 tablespoons dried bread crumbs
¼ cup onion or shallot, finely chopped
1 garlic clove, pressed
1 tablespoon olive oil
1 red bell pepper, chopped
1 jalapeño, chopped
2 tablespoons capers, drained, rinsed and finely chopped
2 tablespoons Dijon mustard
2 tablespoons chopped parsley

1. Sweat the onion, garlic, and red bell pepper in the olive oil, about 5 to 10 minutes.
2. Cut the salmon into 1-inch pieces and pulse grind briefly in a food processor. Don't grind crab meat, but keep it in large pieces until you are ready to form the patties.
3. For salmon cakes, combine the ground salmon with all of the rest of the ingredients except the oil and pulse mix. Form into cakes and refrigerate for at least one hour.
4. For crab cakes, pulse mix all of the ingredients except for the crab and oil. Gently combine the crab meat with the mixed vegetables and form into patties, keeping the large pieces of crab intact. Form into patties and refrigerate for at least one hour
5. Sauté in a small amount of olive oil in a heavy skillet, turning once, about 4 minutes per side.

Makes 4 large or 8 small cakes
220 calories per small cake and 440 calories per large cake, 11.2 g total fat per small cake (46 percent of total calories), 1.7 g saturated, 6.8 g monounsaturated, 2.6 g polyunsaturated, 37 mg cholesterol, 125 mg sodium, 0.6 g fiber

## Codfish Cakes

If upscale restaurants specialize in salmon or crab cakes, codfish cakes arose from more humble origins. My grandmother referred to the codfish aristocracy with disdain, which worried me, because codfish cakes appeared regularly on our menu. I still like them; so do our grandchildren.

1 pound cod, cut into 1-inch pieces
1 packet (8-ounce) of powdered potatoes
1 cup of dried nonfat milk
¼ onion, finely chopped
1 large garlic clove, pressed
1 tablespoon olive oil
¼ cup of egg substitute
1 teaspoon dry mustard
1 teaspoon Worcestershire sauce
4 or 5 sprigs of parsley
1 ½ cups water or vegetable broth

1. Place the cod, egg substitute, mustard, Worcestershire sauce, and parsley in a food processor and mince.
2. Sweat the onion and garlic for 10 minutes and add the water and dried milk. Heat almost to a boil and stir in the powdered potatoes.
3. Add the potato mix to a food processor and mince all of the ingredients.
4. Form into cakes and bake on a greased pan at 375° F for about 30 minutes, or sauté in olive oil.
5. Serve with the mustard or caper sauce found at the beginning of the chapter.

Makes 4 large or 8 small cakes
175 calories per small cake and 350 calories per large cake, 4.1 g total fat per small cake (11 percent of calories), 0.6 g saturated, 2.6 g monounsaturated, 0.5 g polyunsaturated. 12 mg cholesterol, 500 mg sodium, 1.2 g fiber

# *Poultry*

## Mediterranean Chicken, two versions

These variations of chicken cacciatore are hardy and satisfying, yet low in calories. They are not a ragout, because the chicken is sautéed instead of simmered in a stew. The result is fresher and more tender chicken. The first version has North African spices, while version two is more typically Sicilian. Cut the red peppers in quarters, and then place them under the broiler for about 10 minutes to blacken and blister the skin. Cover them with aluminum foil to trap the steam while they cool, and then you can easily peel off the skin before slicing them. Serve the North African version with whole wheat couscous and the Sicilian version with whole -wheat spaghetti.

4 chicken breasts
4 Roma tomatoes diced or one 14 ½-ounce can of tomatoes
2 red bell peppers, seeded, roasted, peeled, and chopped
¼ cup ketchup or tomato paste
1 onion, chopped
3 cloves garlic, pressed
1 tablespoon olive oil
2 tablespoons flour for dusting the chicken
½ teaspoon Cajun seasoning
1 green onion sliced or 3 springs parsley
4 cups of cooked whole grain spaghetti or couscous.

North African version
- 1 teaspoon cumin
- ¼ teaspoon black pepper
- ¼ teaspoon cayenne
- 1 bay leaf

Sicilian version

1 teaspoon oregano
1 teaspoon minced fresh thyme
2 sprigs of parsley, finely chopped
½ cup black olives pitted
¼ cup dry white wine
1 lemon for juice

1. Sweat the onion and garlic for about 10 minutes.
2. Add the roasted bell peppers, tomatoes, ketchup, and ingredients from either version. Simmer for about 15 minutes covered. Add ¼ cup of chicken broth or water if you use fresh Roma tomatoes.
3. Dry the chicken breasts with paper towels and dust with flour and Cajun seasoning in a plastic bag. Sauté for about 7 to 8 minutes per side. Remove and cover with aluminum foil to finish cooking.
4. Pour the tomato and pepper sauce into the fry pan and stir up the brown chicken residue.
5. Slice the chicken across the grain in ¼-inch slices. Spoon the sauce on the spaghetti or couscous and arrange the chicken slices on top. Garnish with green onions or minced parsley.

Serves 4
450 calories per serving including the couscous or spaghetti, 500 calories with olives, 4.3 g total fat (9 percent of calories), 0.3 g saturated, 3.1 g monounsaturated, 0.7 g polyunsaturated, 73 mg cholesterol, 340 mg sodium, 3.5 g fiber

## Spanish Chicken with Red Bell Peppers

In this version of Mediterranean chicken, skip the tomatoes and use lots of red bell peppers. The sherry and orange juice give it a Spanish flavor modified by a little Cajun seasoning when you sauté the chicken. Cut the red peppers in quarters, and then place them under the broiler for about 10 minutes to blacken and blister the skin. Cover them with aluminum foil to trap the steam while they cool, and then you can easily peel off the skin before slicing them. The result is fresh pimento.

4 chicken breasts
4 red bell peppers cut in ½-inch strips
1 cup black olives, coarsely chopped
1 onion, chopped
4 garlic cloves, pressed
1 tablespoon olive oil
2 tablespoons flour for dusting the chicken
1 teaspoon Cajun seasoning
¼ teaspoon cayenne
1 teaspoon fresh thyme
¼ cup of sherry
¼ cup of chicken stock
1 tablespoon fresh orange juice
4 cups of cooked whole grain rice, couscous, or whole wheat pasta

1. Dry the chicken breasts with paper towels and dust with flour and Cajun seasoning. Sauté for about 7 to 8 minutes per side. Remove and cover with aluminum foil.
2. Sweat the onion and garlic in the same frying pan for about 10 minutes stirring up the brown chicken residue.
3. Add the olives, sherry, chicken stock, orange juice, and spices, and simmer for about 2 or 3 minutes.
4. Slice the chicken across the grain in ¼-inch slices and arrange on top of the whole grain rice. Arrange the olives around the chicken, add the red bell peppers and sauce, and garnish with green onions or minced parsley.

Serves 4
460 calories per serving with whole grain rice, 10 g total fat (35 percent of calories), 0.9 g saturated, 8.5 g monounsaturated, 0.9 g polyunsaturated, 70 mg cholesterol, 530 mg sodium, 6.2 g fiber

## Roast Chicken

This was one of Sue's favorite Sunday dinners when she was growing up, although she has embellished her grandmother's recipe with fresh herbs. She varies them using fresh rosemary, tarragon, and lavender from her garden. Carving the roasted chicken at the table makes holiday dinners a nostalgic event. Serve it with Dutch mash or nutmeg-flavored mashed potatoes and a green vegetable.

5 pound roasting hen
2 carrots in ¾-inch chunks
1 onion, chopped
2 cloves garlic, pressed
1 lemon cut in half
1 cup chicken broth
1 cup fresh herbs: choose rosemary, tarragon, or lavender

1. Preheat oven to 425° F.
2. Place carrots and onions in a roasting pan, and put the garlic, two half lemons, and ½ cup herbs into the cavity of the chicken. Put the chicken on top of the bed of carrots and onions, and roast for 1 ½ hours.
3. Remove the chicken from the pan and put aside, scooping out the lemon and herbs.
4. Put the lemon, herbs, and juices from the cavity in the roasting pan with the vegetables, and add the chicken broth and the other ½ cup of fresh herbs. Bring to a boil and scrape the pan to blend all of the roasting juices into a sauce.
5. Strain the sauce and discard the vegetables, herbs, and lemons. Put the strained sauce in a gravy separator to remove the fat. (A gravy separator looks like a small watering can with the spout attached near the bottom of the can. Since fat rises to the top, you can pour nonfat sauce from the spout.)
6. Put the defatted sauce into a saucepan and keep warm. Apply high heat to concentrate it, if necessary. Save any juices from carving the chicken and add to the sauce.

Serves 6 to 8
225 calories per serving, 4.5 g total fat (22 percent of calories), 1.2 g saturated, 1.7 g monounsaturated, 0.9 g polyunsaturated, 105 mg cholesterol, 100 mg sodium, 0 g fiber

## Broiled Chicken with a Lemon and Garlic Marinade

Marinating enhances the flavor and tenderizes the chicken. This simple recipe has many variations and works with many of the pasta and vegetable recipes later in the book.

4 chicken breasts
1 tablespoon olive oil
2 garlic cloves, pressed
¼ cup lemon juice
2 bay leaves

1. Place the chicken breasts, lemon juice, olive oil, garlic, and bay leaves in a plastic bag and marinate in the refrigerator for at least 2 hours.
2. Broil the chicken breasts for 6 minutes on the first side, then turn and baste with the marinade. Broil the second side for 4 to 6 minutes.
3. Remove and cover with aluminum foil for 10 minutes before slicing across the grain into ¼ strips.

Serves 4
200 calories per serving, 4.0 g total fat (13 percent of calories), 0.4 g saturated, 1.8 g monounsaturated, 0.6 g polyunsaturated, 75 mg cholesterol, 100 mg sodium. 0 fiber

## Lemon Chicken à la North Conway

Hikers and skiers in a lodge in North Conway, New Hampshire, enjoy this stir-fried variation of chicken cacciatore. Mediterranean and Cantonese cuisine are migrating north. Serve it over any type of whole wheat pasta.

2 chicken breasts
12 medium mushrooms, halved
2 Roma tomatoes in wedges
½ green bell pepper in ¾-inch chunks
1 shallot, chopped
1 clove garlic, pressed
1 tablespoon olive oil
¼ teaspoon nutmeg
¼ cup lemon juice
¼ cup Sherry
Flour to coat chicken
½ pound whole wheat spaghetti
4 or 5 sprigs of parsley, chopped

1. Cut the chicken breasts into 1-inch cubes, coat with flour and nutmeg, and sauté in olive oil for about 5 minutes. Set aside.
2. In the same frying pan, add more oil and sauté the mushrooms. Set aside.
3. Sweat the garlic and shallots for about 5 minutes, and then add the green pepper for another 5 minutes.
4. Add back the tomatoes, chicken pieces, and mushrooms, plus any remaining flour, and pour the lemon juice and wine over them. Bring to a boil for about a minute, cover, and turn off the heat.
5. Serve over pasta and garnish with parsley.

Serves 2
380 calories per serving, 10 g total fat (23 percent of calories), 2.0 g saturated, 8.6 g monounsaturated, 0.9 g polyunsaturated, 36 mg cholesterol, 500 mg sodium, 5 g fiber

## Irish Italian Stew

Who ever heard of Italian food with dumplings? Irish Italian stew originated in the melting-pot neighborhood in New York where Sue's grandmother grew up. She liked dumplings, but not spaghetti. So in her house, you got your chicken cacciatore with potatoes and dumplings. Even her Italian friends liked it, and now you can enjoy this all-American delight in big soup bowls with San Francisco whole wheat sourdough bread.

1 chicken (3 pounds) cut in pieces
3 carrots in ¾-inch chunks
2 potatoes in ¾-inch chunks
1 onion, chopped
1 stalk celery in ¾-inch slices
3 cloves of garlic, pressed
1 tablespoon olive oil
1 large can tomato sauce
1 teaspoon oregano
½ teaspoon black pepper
1 bay leaf
Dumplings
  1 cup cracker meal
  ¼ cup egg substitute
  2 tablespoons parmesan cheese

1. Dry the chicken pieces with paper towels and brown in olive oil in an ovenproof casserole on top of the stove. Remove and set aside.
2. Sweat the onions and celery in the drippings for about 10 minutes.
3. Add the rest of the vegetables, herbs, and tomato sauce, and bring to a boil. Then add back the chicken pieces and any accumulated juices. Cover the casserole and bake in a preheated oven at 400° F for 1 ½ hours.
4. To make dumplings, mix the cracker meal, egg substitute, and cheese, and form into 1-inch balls that will seem stiff. Add to the boiling liquid in the casserole, recover, and cook an additional 15 minutes.
5. Serve in soup bowls with whole grain bread and a green salad.

Serves 6
325 calories per serving, 8.4 g total fat (23 percent of calories), 2.7 g saturated, 3.5 g monounsaturated, 1.6 g polyunsaturated, 90 mg cholesterol, 360 mg sodium, 4.0 g fiber

## Chicken with Grapes (or Cherries)

Fruit dresses up the appearance of ordinary broiled or sautéed chicken and brings out a flavor entirely different from savory dishes. Grapes, cherries, and many other types of fruit work just as well by varying the type of jam. When in doubt, use apricot jam. Serve it with steamed brown rice mixed with garden peas and a small amount of olive oil.

2 half, boneless, skinless chicken breasts
1 tablespoon olive oil
¼ cup orange marmalade (use apricot or cherry jam for cherries)
1 cup of Thompson seedless grapes
2 tablespoons lemon juice
Flour to coat chicken
¼ teaspoon black pepper
Watercress sprigs

1. Dry the chicken with paper towels and coat with a thin layer of flour containing the black pepper.
2. Sauté the chicken on medium high in a large frying pan, about 5 minutes per side. Remove and cover with aluminum foil for another 10 minutes.
3. Deglaze the pan with the marmalade and lemon juice, adding a small amount of water if needed. Add the grapes for the last minute.
4. Slice the chicken breasts across the grain into ¼-inch slices and garnish with watercress sprigs.
5. Arrange the chicken slices on each plate, drizzle the deglazed sauce on top and arrange the grapes on the side.

Serves 4
300 calories per serving plus rice, 4.0 g total fat (11 percent of calories), 0.5 g saturated, 2.2 g monounsaturated, 0.5 g polyunsaturated, 73 mg cholesterol, 100 mg sodium, 1.6 g fiber

## Chicken Curry

British colonists brought curried dishes back to London from India in the nineteenth century, and now you can find them all over the world. In the railroad stations in Japan, they don't sell hot dogs, and they don't sell tempura either; but you can find chicken curry.

2 chicken breasts cut into 1-inch cubes
1 large onion sliced with the grain
2 ½ tablespoons curry powder
1 tablespoon chili powder
1 cup nonfat milk
2 tablespoons flour
1 tablespoons safflower or canola oil

1. Dry the chicken breasts with paper towels, cube, and brown in the cooking oil. Remove and set aside.
2. In the same pan, sauté the onions until golden.
3. Meanwhile, whisk the spices and flour into nonfat milk, and pour the mix on the golden onions, scraping the chicken and onion remnants from bottom of the pan.
4. Return the chicken to the pan along with any chicken juices. Stir and simmer an additional 2 or 3 minutes.
5. Serve the chicken with brown rice, fruit, and chutney.

Serves 4
200 calories per serving, 7.3 g total fat (28 percent of calories), 1.0 g saturated, 4.1 g monounsaturated, 2.1 g polyunsaturated, 56 mg cholesterol, 80 mg sodium, 0.6 g fiber

## Chicken and Dumplings

Sue's great-grandmother from the Isle of Wight contributed this one. Sue added the wine to the recipe about a century later. Chicken and dumplings is a good use of leftover roast chicken or turkey, but fresh chicken breasts sautéed work well, too. Sue gets high praise from our grandchildren for chicken and dumplings.

1 pound chicken breasts, or leftover chicken, cubed and sautéed
3 large carrots cut cross-section
3 small red potatoes in ¾-inch cubes (peeling not necessary)
1 small rutabaga in ¾-inch cubes
1 cup peas, lima beans, or string beans in 1-inch lengths
3 cups liquid: chicken broth, or water with packaged turkey gravy
¾ cup white wine
Dumplings:
  1 cup corn meal
  1 cup oatmeal
  1 cup flour
  1 ½ cups nonfat milk
  1 tablespoon baking powder
  ½ cup chopped flat parsley
  1 teaspoon black pepper

1. Boil carrots, rutabaga, and potatoes in a large pot for 10 minutes. Drain, but retain some of the water.
2. Add the chicken, the green vegetables, the wine, and 3 cups of chicken broth, or water with packaged turkey gravy. You can use some of the water from the boiled root vegetables to bring the level to ½ inch above the vegetables and chicken. Bring to a boil.
3. Mix the dumpling ingredients together in a bowl. The consistency should be slightly thinner than for biscuits.
4. Spoon the mix into the boiling chicken and vegetables, cover, and simmer for 15 minutes.

Serves 6
400 calories per serving, 4.3 g total fat (10 percent of calories), 0.6 g saturated, 0.7 g monounsaturated, 0.7 g polyunsaturated, 74 mg cholesterol, 440 mg sodium, 5.3 g fiber

## Mexican Chili Mole with Ground Turkey

Chocolate chili con carne with ground turkey practically requires Sue's corn bread in the bread section of the book. Add a tomato and lettuce salad.

1 pound ground turkey breast
2 cups cooked red kidney beans
1 onion, chopped
3 cloves garlic, pressed
1 small can tomato paste
1 can (14 ½-ounce) diced tomatoes
1 tablespoon molasses
¼ teaspoon cayenne
2 tablespoons unsweetened cocoa
1 teaspoon paprika
1 teaspoon cumin
½ teaspoon oregano

1. Fry the onion on low in small amount of olive oil for 10 minutes, browning the onion slightly.
2. Crumble the turkey and garlic into the pan and sauté until the turkey is completely cooked.
3. Stir in the rest of the ingredients together with about 1 cup of water and bring to a boil. Cover and simmer for about 30 minutes. Add more water if necessary.
4. Serve with brown rice or corn bread.

Serves 4
260 calories per serving, 8.0 g total fat (27 percent of calories), 2.0 g saturated, 4.2 g monounsaturated, 1.3 g polyunsaturated, 65 mg cholesterol, 700 mg sodium, 7.3 g fiber

## Apple Turkey Loaf

Bake this turkey loaf on the weekend and serve it throughout the week. Heat and serve it with mashed potatoes and a green vegetable, or serve it cold in a sandwich or salad.

2 ½ pounds ground turkey breast
1 apple with skin, cored and chopped
1 ½ onion, chopped
1 clove garlic, pressed
1 tablespoon olive oil
1 cup fine dry bread crumbs
¼ cup ketchup
2 tablespoons Worcestershire sauce
1 teaspoon *herbes de Provence*
1 teaspoon black pepper

1. Sauté onion, garlic, and apples over medium heat, constantly stirring, for about 7 minutes.
2. Allow to cool, then combine in a bowl with all the other ingredients.
3. Mold in a 9-inch loaf pan and top with extra ketchup and bake at 340° F for about 2 hours.
4. Serve hot, or refrigerate and serve cold.

Serves 6
240 calories per serving, 3 g total fat (13 percent of calories), 0.7 g saturated, 1.6 g monounsaturated, 0.5 g polyunsaturated, 75 mg cholesterol, 185 mg sodium, 1.6 g fiber

# *Pasta, Rice, and Couscous*

## Spaghetti Sauce with Sun-Dried Tomatoes, Olives, and Capers

Residents of the Island of Crete would recognize this hardy recipe, as would all Sicilians and Neapolitans. Sue's grandmother could never match real Mediterranean spaghetti sauce, but Sue can.

2 or 3 pounds tomatoes, or one 28-ounce can of tomatoes
1 small can tomato paste
2 tablespoons sun-dried tomatoes in oil, chopped
1 cup pitted black olives
1 onion, chopped
3 garlic cloves, crushed
1 small carrot, chopped
4 tablespoons capers
1 tablespoon olive oil
¼ teaspoon cayenne
½ teaspoon oregano
½ cup parsley minced
1 pound whole wheat spaghetti cooked

1. Sweat onion, garlic, carrots, and sun-dried tomatoes in olive oil for about 10 minutes or until caramelized.
2. Add the tomatoes, tomato paste, oregano, and cayenne, and simmer for 40 minutes. Blend with an electric handheld blender.
3. Turn off heat and add capers, parsley, and black olives.
4. Serve over spaghetti.

Serves 8
270 calories per serving with spaghetti, 7.5 g total fat (21 percent of calories), 0.3 g saturated, 6.9 g monounsaturated, 0.2 g polyunsaturated, 0 cholesterol, 450 mg sodium, 1.8 g fiber

## Whole Wheat Spaghetti with Lemon and Pepper Sauce

The lemon and pepper sauce makes a nice upgrade from ordinary boiled pasta to be served with many Mediterranean dishes, or just with a salad.

1 tablespoon olive oil
2 large garlic cloves, crushed
2 lemons for juice and zest
1 teaspoon ground black pepper
¼ teaspoon red pepper flakes
¾ pound whole wheat spaghetti, cooked

1. Sweat the garlic, black pepper, and red pepper flakes in olive oil for 2 minutes, taking care not to burn the garlic.
2. Remove from the heat, combine, and toss with the hot spaghetti and lemon zest and juice.

Serves 4
200 calories per serving, 7.0 g total fat (30 percent of calories), 0.4 g saturated fat, 5.9 g monounsaturated fat, 0.8 g polyunsaturated fat, 0 g cholesterol, 130 mg sodium, 1 g fiber

## Pasta with Seafood in an Orange Sauce

Almost any seafood works well with this Mediterranean dish, especially white fish, calamari, shrimp, and scallops. Cut the red bell peppers in quarters, and then place them under the broiler for about 10 minutes to blacken and blister the skin. Cover them with aluminum foil to trap the steam while they cool, and then you can easily peel off the skin before slicing them.

2 ½ pounds scallops, calamari, shrimp, cod, sablefish, orange roughy, halibut or sea bass, in any combination
3 red bell peppers
½ onion, chopped
4 garlic cloves, pressed
1 tablespoon olive oil
¼ cup orange juice, freshly squeezed
2 medium oranges for zest
¼ teaspoon hot pepper flakes
⅔ pound whole wheat spaghetti

1. Boil the pasta and set aside.
2. Blister and peel the red bell peppers as above, and slice them into long thin strips.
3. In a large pot, sweat the onion, garlic, and hot pepper flakes in the olive oil for about 10 minutes.
4. Add the shrimp, calamari, and fish, and cook on low an additional 3 minutes.
5. Stir in the orange juice, zest, and red bell pepper strips and toss together with the pasta.

Serves 6
350 calories per serving, 7.0 g total fat (18 percent of calories), 0.2 g saturated, 5.2 g monounsaturated, 0.3 g polyunsaturated, 50 mg cholesterol, 240 mg sodium, 1.7 g fiber

## Risotto with Tomatoes and Butternut Squash

Steam the brown rice using plain water in a rice cooker, and add a small amount of chicken broth later for flavor; rice steamed in broth develops a mushy surface and a hard core. This version can stand alone as a main course, or serve it with steamed shellfish or thin slices of broiled chicken breast.

4 Roma tomatoes, crushed and drained
2 cups of butternut squash, chopped into ½-inch chunks
1 medium onion, chopped
2 garlic cloves, pressed
1 tablespoon olive oil
1 ½ cups brown rice, dry
¾ cup chicken or vegetable broth
¼ teaspoon cinnamon
½ teaspoon sugar
¼ teaspoon cayenne
½ teaspoon oregano
½ cup parsley or cilantro, chopped

1. Steam the brown rice in 4 ½ cups of water in a rice cooker.
2. Sweat the onion and garlic in a small amount of olive oil for about 10 minutes.
3. Add the butternut squash, cayenne, oregano, and cinnamon and sauté on medium-high for another 10 minutes.
4. Add the tomatoes, chicken broth, and sugar, and simmer for about 20 minutes or until the squash is cooked.
5. Combine with the brown rice and mix in the parsley or cilantro.

Serves 4
160 calories per serving, 2.4 g total fat (14 percent of calories), 0.2 g saturated, 1.7 g monounsaturated, 0.2 g polyunsaturated, 0 cholesterol, 220 mg sodium, 1.7 g fiber

## Whole Wheat Couscous

Using whole wheat couscous doubles the amount of fiber. This recipe is simpler than the North African version, but it works well as a side dish with many chicken and fish dishes.

8 ounces whole wheat couscous
1 carrot, diced
½ rutabaga, diced
1 tablespoon olive oil
1 tablespoon flat leaf parsley, minced
2 cups water

1. Boil the vegetables covered in 2 cups of water for about 20 minutes until cooked, but still firm.
2. Stir in the couscous and olive oil and turn off heat.
3. Cover and let stand for 15 minutes.
4. Fluff with the parsley and serve.

Serves 5
280 calories per serving, 3.5 g total fat (11 percent of total), 0.3 g saturated, 2.6 g monounsaturated, 0.3 g polyunsaturated, 0 mg cholesterol, 6.0 g fiber, 10 mg sodium

## Whole Wheat Couscous Steamed in Chicken Stock and Milk

The powdered milk in this Moroccan version adds body to the couscous, and you can avoid the film that forms on the surface of boiled fresh milk. Preparation time is only about 5 minutes.

⅓ cup whole wheat couscous
2 tablespoons dry nonfat milk
⅔ cup chicken stock
1 teaspoon olive oil

1. Dissolve the nonfat milk in the cold chicken stock and add the olive oil.
2. Heat to boiling in a microwave, remove, add the couscous, and cover for 5 minutes.
3. Fluff the couscous with a fork and serve on a platter.

Serves 2
230 calories per serving, 3.5 g total fat (13 percent of total), 0.3 g saturated, 2.6 g monounsaturated, 0.3 g polyunsaturated, 0 mg cholesterol, 5.0 g fiber, 10 mg sodium (more if commercial chicken broth is used)

## North African Couscous

Savory couscous can serve as a main course, but it can also accompany other Mediterranean dishes, such as the Broiled Chicken in a Garlic Marinade in the poultry section. Many Parisian restaurants offer a similar version.

6 ounces dry whole wheat couscous
1 cup butternut squash diced in 1-inch chunks
1 onion, chopped
2 carrots, diced in 1-inch chunks
2 small zucchini diced in 1-inch chunks
½ red bell pepper, chopped
½ cup dried chickpeas, soaked overnight and boiled until tender
1 tablespoon olive oil
1 cup chicken stock
1 teaspoon cumin
¼ teaspoon black pepper
⅛ to ¼ teaspoon cayenne according to taste
3 or 4 sprigs of parsley minced
12 orange slices

1. Place the squash, onions, carrots, red bell pepper, and zucchini in a plastic bag and shake with the olive oil and pepper.
2. Roast the vegetables in the oven for 1 hour at 375° F, turning once or twice.
3. Add the cumin, and pepper to the chicken stock and bring to a boil.
4. Add the couscous to the stock, cover, and turn off the heat. Allow to stand for 15 minutes.
5. Mix in the roasted vegetables, chickpeas, and parsley with the couscous.
6. Serve with nonfat yogurt and garnish with orange slices, or layer thin slices of broiled chicken on top.

Serves 4
210 calories per serving, 4.2 g total fat (18 percent of calories), 0.5 g saturated fat, 2.8 g monounsaturated fat, 0.6 g polyunsaturated fat, 0 cholesterol, 100 mg sodium, 6.4 g fiber

## Israeli Couscous

The Israelis make couscous from the same semolina found in the North African version, but in Israel each grain is larger and softer like pasta.

1 cup Israeli couscous, dry
2 cups chicken broth
1 teaspoon olive oil
1 tablespoon chopped parsley
1 teaspoon black pepper

1. Bring the broth, olive oil, and pepper to a boil.
2. Add the couscous, cover, and simmer for 15 minutes stirring every 5 minutes. Add water if the couscous begins to stick.
3. Mix in parsley and serve.

Serves 4
150 calories per serving, 0.2 g total fat (1 percent of calories), 0 g saturated, 0 g monounsaturated, 0.1 g polyunsaturated, 0 cholesterol, 2.0 g fiber, 7 mg sodium

## Spelt Berry Pilaf

Spelt berries date from antiquity and are a primitive relative of wheat. Austrians have grown them for centuries, and now specialty groceries and some supermarkets in the United States sell them. Together with a small amount of wild rice, they make a hardy pilaf with a nutty flavor that enhances any principle dish. If you can't find the spelt berries, substitute barley and call it Scottish.

1 cup spelt berries
½ cup wild rice
3 cups water
¼ cup chicken broth
¼ cup chopped cilantro and green onions

1. Cook the mix of spelt berries, wild rice, and water in a rice cooker.
2. When finished cooking, mix in the chicken broth and herbs, and fluff with a fork.

Serves 4
200 calories per serving, 1.6 g total fat (7 percent of total), 0.1 g saturated, 0.9 g monounsaturated, 0.5 g polyunsaturated, 0 mg cholesterol, 5.0 g fiber, 20 mg sodium

## Jambalaya

Just as Chinese immigrants in San Francisco invented chow mein and chop suey from leftovers, the Cajuns around New Orleans invented jambalaya. They brought their French language with them, including the word for ham, *jambon*. Jambalaya means a ham stew. However, ham was not always available, so now you can find shrimp, oysters, Andouille sausage, chicken, beef, and many kinds of fish in jambalaya. Don't forget the cayenne.

¾ pound raw shrimp, peeled
¾ pound calamari
1 chicken breast cut into ¾-inch pieces
1 onion, chopped
4 cloves garlic, pressed
1 can (14.5-ounce) of diced tomatoes
1 red bell pepper, chopped
1 tablespoon olive oil
1½ cups of dry brown rice
½ cup of chicken stock
1 teaspoon cumin
½ teaspoon thyme
½ teaspoon allspice
¼ teaspoon cayenne
¼ teaspoon cloves
¼ teaspoon black pepper

1. Steam the rice in 4 ½ cups of water in a rice cooker
2. Sweat the onions, bell pepper, and garlic in the olive oil in a large pot.
3. Add the chicken to the pot together with all of the spices, and sauté for about 5 minutes.
4. Stir in the tomatoes with their juice and a small amount of chicken stock if needed. Bring to a boil and cook for another 3 minutes.
5. Add the shrimp and calamari, cover and cook for one minute, and turn off the heat. Allow to stand for five minutes to finish cooking.
6. Mix in the rice and serve.

Serves 6
320 calories per serving, 5.4 g total fat (17 percent of calories), 1.0 g saturated fat, 2.5 g monounsaturated fat, 1.2 g polyunsaturated fat, 41 mg cholesterol, 160 mg sodium, 2.5 g fiber

## Whole Grain Pizza

Homemade pizza has no limits for topping combinations. Here we use green bell peppers, artichoke hearts, spinach, and black olives. This recipe also contains a fraction of the oil and calories of commercial pizza. You won't ever want commercial pizza again after tasting the whole grain crust.

1 packet of yeast
¼ teaspoon sugar
1½ cups flour
1½ cups whole-wheat flour
½ cup corn meal
¼ cup olive oil
2 cloves garlic, pressed
1 cup lukewarm water
Topping
  1 can (14½-ounce) diced tomatoes, drained
  ½ green bell pepper, chopped
  ½ package frozen artichoke hearts
  1 large handful of fresh spinach leaves
  10 or 12 black olives cut in half
  1 teaspoon oregano
  1 cup nonfat feta cheese

1. Dissolve the yeast in 1 cup warm water and add all of the dough ingredients. Adjust with more flour or water to make a firm dough.
2. Knead on a dough hook and let rise for 1½ hours.
3. Spread the dough on a pizza stone. Apply the garlic on the dough with a knife and add the topping.
4. Bake at 450° F for 30 to 40 minutes depending upon the amount of topping.

Makes one 15-inch pizza, 8 slices
250 calories per ⅛ slice, 8.4 g total fat (32 percent of calories), 0.5 g saturated, 7.1 g monounsaturated, 0.8 g polyunsaturated, 0 cholesterol, 300 mg sodium, 6.2 g fiber

# *Asian Food*

## Lingcod in Black Bean Sauce

The restaurant Jing Jing in Palo Alto has served a similar dish for more than half a century, and it has been my favorite for almost as long. You can substitute orange roughy, halibut, or sablefish for the lingcod.

1½ pound lingcod in 1- or 2-inch pieces
¼ pound snow peas or sweet edible pea pods
½ red bell pepper in ¾-inch strips
2 jalapeño peppers, seeded and chopped
2 carrots, sliced diagonally
1 stalk of celery, sliced crosswise
¼ pound mushrooms, halved
4-inch piece ginger root, peeled and chopped
1 tablespoon sesame oil
Sauce:
  2 tablespoons black bean garlic sauce
  2 tablespoons sweet sherry
  2 tablespoons low-sodium soy sauce
  1 tablespoon corn starch
  1 cup water
  2 green onions, chopped

1. Stir-fry ginger and mushrooms in 1 tablespoon sesame oil until the liquid disappears.
2. Add carrots, celery, and peppers and stir-fry for about 3 minutes. Add peas for 1 additional minute.
3. Add the ling cod together with the sauce made from the last 6 ingredients. Steam the cod in the liquid for about 2 to 3 minutes and serve.

Makes 4 servings
200 calories per serving, 0.7 g total fat (5 percent of calories), 0.1 g saturated, 0.2 g monounsaturated, 0.2 g polyunsaturated, 20 mg cholesterol, 700 mg sodium, 2.4 g fiber

## Tofu with Mushrooms and Snow Peas

You can stir-fry tofu and mushrooms with almost any garden vegetable, such as snow peas, broccoli, or fresh tomatoes, and serve it over rice for a complete meal. Preparation time from start to finish is only about 20 minutes.

½ pound mushrooms sliced (any variety)
1 package (14-ounce) of firm tofu, cut into ¾-inch cubes
1-inch peeled ginger, chopped
3 green onions, sliced crosswise
½ pound snow peas
Sauce:
 1 tablespoon cornstarch
 2 tablespoons low-sodium soy sauce
 1 cup water

1. Stir-fry the mushrooms and ginger in sesame oil. Remove to a side dish and add more oil to the skillet.
2. Stir-fry the tofu until golden brown on all sides and add back in the mushrooms and ginger. Add the snow peas.
3. Combine and whisk the sauce ingredients and pour over tofu, mushrooms, and snow peas, heating and stirring carefully until the sauce thickens.

Makes 4 servings
225 calories per serving plus rice, 11.0 g total fat (44 percent of calories), 1.6 g saturated, 2.4 g monounsaturated, 6.2 g polyunsaturated, 0 cholesterol, 480 mg sodium, 2.9 g fiber

## Tofu, Spinach, and Noodles in a Peanut Butter Sauce

The preparation takes only a few minutes for this simple variation of a classic Szechuan dish. Serve it for lunch or supper as a one-dish meal.

14 ounces extra firm tofu, cut into ¾-inch cubes
½ pound whole wheat spaghetti or Chinese rice noodles
8 ounce package of spinach
2 green onions, sliced
Sauce:
  1 tablespoon peanut butter
  1 tablespoon distilled vinegar
  2 tablespoons sesame oil
  2 tablespoons low-sodium soy sauce
  ¼ teaspoon red pepper flakes

1. Combine the sauce ingredients in a bowl and heat to boiling in the microwave. Whisk to blend in the peanut butter.
2. Boil the noodles in water adding the tofu during the last 2 minutes.
3. Place the spinach in a colander in the sink and pour the boiling water with the noodle and tofu mix on top to steam the spinach. Further cooking of the spinach isn't necessary.
4. Heat the sauce ingredients in the microwave and whisk until smooth.
5. Place into a serving dish and mix in the sauce.

Makes 4 servings of tofu and 4 servings of pasta or noodles
450 calories per serving, 18.6 g total fat (38 percent of calories), 2.8 g saturated, 5.6 g monounsaturated, 9.2 g polyunsaturated, 275 mg sodium, 7.0 g fiber

## Spicy Green Beans and Nonfat Turkey Sausage

This delicious quick-prep dish appears on many Chinese restaurant menus, except our recipe has fewer calories. We prefer the foot-long green beans.

1 pound green beans (French, Italian, or foot-long Chinese string beans)
½ pound nonfat spicy turkey or chicken sausage (see Tips and Tricks)
½ tablespoon sesame oil
1 jalapeño, chopped, or ¼ teaspoon cayenne
Sauce:
- 3 tablespoons low-sodium soy sauce
- ½ tablespoon corn starch
- 1 teaspoon sugar
- ½ cup water

1. Sauté meat and chopped pepper, but use only ½ of the seeds and ½ of the lining membrane of the pepper.
2. Add the green beans and sauté for an additional 3 minutes.
3. Whisk the sauce ingredients and pour over the beans and meat. Stir and cook on high until it thickens and serve.

Makes 4 servings
115 calories per serving plus rice, 3.9 g total fat (38 percent of calories), 1.0 g saturated, 2.9 g monounsaturated, 3.0 g polyunsaturated, 11 mg cholesterol, 240 mg sodium, 2.0 g fiber

## Mushrooms, Cabbage, and Bamboo Shoots with Noodles

Cantonese spaghetti with vegetables existed before Marco Polo imported pasta into Italy. We substitute regular whole wheat spaghetti for the more authentic rice noodles.

½ pound whole wheat spaghetti
1 small chicken breast, shredded
½ small cabbage, shredded
1 can bamboo shoots, drained and chopped
1 cup fresh mushrooms in pieces
1 carrot, shredded
1 tablespoon sesame oil
Sauce:
  1 tablespoon dry sherry
  2 tablespoons corn starch
  3 tablespoons low-sodium soy sauce
  1½ cups chicken stock or water

1. Steam the noodles (about 9 minutes), and then fry them with a small amount of sesame oil in a skillet over medium heat. When the first side is golden, flip the noodles and fry the other side.
2. In another skillet, stir-fry the mushrooms in a small amount of sesame oil until the liquid is gone.
3. Add meat, cabbage, carrots, and bamboo shoots, and stir-fry until the meat is cooked.
4. Combine and whisk the sauce ingredients and pour over the meat and cabbage mix. Heat and stir until thickened.
5. Serve the chicken and vegetables on top of the fried noodles.

Makes 2 portions
240 calories per serving, 8.8 g total fat (33 percent of calories), 1.4 g saturated, 3.1 g monounsaturated, 3.4 g polyunsaturated, 190 mg sodium, 3.8 g fiber

## Sweet and Sour Fish (or Shrimp)

Fresh ginger and snow peas enhance the flavor and color of this classic Chinese dish. Scallops, shrimp, white fish, or chicken all work equally well.

1 pound raw white fish in 1-inch squares (or 1 pound of raw shrimp shelled)
1 sweet red bell pepper cut into ¾-inch squares
1 carrot cut into ¾ inch cubes
½ onion, chopped
1 clove garlic, crushed
1 tablespoon sesame oil
1 can (14 ½-ounce) pineapple chunks
1 teaspoon powdered ginger or 1 tablespoon chopped fresh ginger
¼ cup cilantro, chopped
Sauce:
  ½ cup cider vinegar
  4 tablespoons low-sodium soy sauce
  2 tablespoons ketchup
  2 tablespoons cornstarch
  1 tablespoon dry sherry

1. Stir-fry the onions, peppers, carrots, and garlic in the cooking oil on low for about 12 minutes.
2. Add drained pineapple chunks, but save the liquid for the sauce.
3. Stir-fry for 2 more minutes, then add the sauce and turn up the heat until boiling, stirring until the sauce thickens. Add pineapple juice to obtain the right consistency.
4. Add the fish carefully without breaking it apart stirring gently for 1 minute.
5. Garnish with cilantro and serve.

Makes 4 servings
225 calories per serving, 5.2 g total fat (21 percent of calories), 0.3 g saturated, 0.3 monounsaturated, 0.4 g polyunsaturated, 44 mg cholesterol, 320 mg sodium, 1.7 g fiber

## Egg Foo Yung

Egg foo yung is one of the first Cantonese dishes that Chinese immigrants introduced in the nineteenth century. Some say those immigrants invented it after arriving in California, and that egg foo young is really an American dish. Sue learned it from her Irish grandmother.

8 ounces egg substitute
½ cup cooked chicken or shrimp
½ cup celery, grated
½ cup mushrooms shredded (cut longitudinally)
1 cup bean sprouts
¼ cup fresh onion, shredded
1 teaspoon sherry
¼ teaspoon black pepper
1 tablespoons vegetable oil
Sauce:
  12 ounces chicken broth
  1 teaspoon ketchup
  1 tablespoon low-sodium soy sauce
  2½ tablespoons flour

1. Combine eggs with all of the ingredients except for the sauce.
2. Spoon the mix onto a skillet to make pancakes. Flip when the edges are cooked thoroughly, about 3 or 4 minutes per side. Place onto a serving dish.
3. Combine the sauce ingredients and beat with a wire whisk. Cook in a microwave until boiling.
4. Pour the sauce over the pancakes.

Makes 4 servings
185 calories per serving, 7.8 g saturated (38 percent of calories), 0.9 g saturated, 5.4 g monounsaturated, 0.8 g polyunsaturated, 18 mg cholesterol, 300 mg sodium, 0.7 g fiber

# *Vegetables*

Many fresh vegetables taste their best raw or steamed. Celery and lettuce have negligible calories, and a serving of steamed spinach, zucchini, or cabbage contains only about fifteen calories. Broccoli, cauliflower, green beans, and tomatoes have less than twenty-five calories per serving. Although the U.S. Department of Agriculture pyramid recommends five servings of vegetables per day for a daily diet of two thousand calories, larger quantities of vegetables add very few calories, especially if you enjoy the vegetables raw or steamed. If instead, you prefer to dress up your vegetables, the recipes that follow are delicious, and most of the calories come from olive oil, which is rich in monounsaturated fat.

## Steamed Spinach with Shallots

Shallots and olive oil enhance plain steamed spinach. Most of the calories come from just ½ tablespoon of olive oil split four ways. That's because one serving of steamed spinach contains only about 10 calories. Try using citrus-flavored olive oil.

1 pound bag washed spinach
2 shallots chopped
½ tablespoon olive oil

1. Sweat the shallots in the olive oil in a large pot for about 5 or 6 minutes.
2. Add the spinach and cover. Heat for 2 or 3 minutes, shaking the pot so that the spinach doesn't stick.
3. Turn off the heat and serve.

Serves 4
35 calories per serving, 2.7 g total fat (72 percent of calories), 0.3 g saturated, 1.9 g monounsaturated, 0.4 g polyunsaturated, 0 cholesterol, 2 mg sodium, 0.3 g fiber

## Baked Tomatoes

Consider baking tomatoes any time the oven is set at a medium temperature for an hour or more, for example, when apple turkey loaf is on the menu. Baked tomatoes are always a treat.

8 or more tomatoes (Roma work well)
1 cup fine dry bread crumbs
2 clove garlic, pressed
2 tablespoon olive oil
1 teaspoon black pepper

1. Cut the tomatoes in half crosswise and place in a banking dish.
2. Drizzle a mix of crushed garlic and olive oil over each tomato half. Sprinkle with pepper and top with the bread crumbs.
3. Bake at 340° F for 1 ½ hours.

Serves 4
75 calories per serving, 7.0 g total fat (80 percent of calories), 0.6 g saturated, 5.2 g monounsaturated, 0.6 g polyunsaturated, 0 cholesterol, 4 mg sodium, 0.7 g fiber

## Three Recipes for French Haricots Verts

French string beans are thinner and more tender than Kentucky Wonder or Blue Lake beans, the most common varieties in American food markets. Consequently, the cooking time is shorter for the French variety. Some French chefs cook the string beans until they are limp; that's a major culinary offense in San Francisco. Try using citrus-flavored olive oil. Don't overcook the beans.

1. String beans with red bell pepper

1 pound French string beans with both ends removed
½ red bell pepper, diced
1 shallot, chopped
1 tablespoon olive oil
¼ teaspoon black pepper

1. Blanch the string beans in a large pot of boiling water for 4 minutes. Drain immediately and immerse in a bowl of cold water to stop the cooking.
2. Sauté the red bell pepper and chopped shallot in the olive oil together with the black pepper until they are slightly browned and fragrant.
3. Just before serving, add the blanched string beans and warm.

2. String beans with lemon and garlic sauce

1 pound French string beans blanched as above
1 tablespoon olive oil
1 clove garlic
1 Meyer lemon for zest and juice

1. Combine the olive oil, garlic, lemon juice, and zest to make a sauce.
2. Mix with the beans just before serving.

3. String beans with toasted almonds

1 pound French string beans blanched as above
1 tablespoon olive oil
½ cup slivered almonds

1. Sauté the almonds in the olive oil for 3 or 4 minutes.
2. Mix with the beans just before serving and warm

Serves 6

About 70 calories per serving for versions one and two, 2.6 g total fat (39 percent of calories), 0.3 g saturated, 1.7 g monounsaturated, 0.4 g polyunsaturated, 0 cholesterol, 2 mg sodium, 1.9 g fiber

For version three, the almonds add 80 calories per serving, 7 g total fat (80 percent of calories), 0.7 g saturated, 4.8 g monounsaturated, 1.6 g polyunsaturated, 0 g cholesterol, 2.0 g fiber, 2 mg sodium

## Braised Bell Peppers, Zucchini, or Green Beans with Tomatoes

Mediterranean cooks add tomatoes to any vegetable, green or otherwise. Don't overcook the green vegetables.

4 small zucchini, or 1 pound flat Italian green beans, or 3 bell peppers in 1-inch pieces
4 Roma tomatoes, sliced
1 large onion, finely chopped
1 large clove of garlic, pressed
1 tablespoon olive oil
1 teaspoon oregano

1. Sweat the onion and garlic in the olive oil for 10 minutes over low heat.
2. Stir-fry the zucchini, green beans, or bell peppers in the onion and garlic mix.
3. Add the tomatoes and oregano.
4. Cover and simmer for about 5 minutes.

Makes 4 servings
100 calories per serving, 3.5 g total fat (51 percent of calories), 0.5 g saturated, 2.6 g monounsaturated, 0.3 g polyunsaturated, 0 cholesterol, 2 mg sodium, 2.6 g fiber

## Red Beans New Orleans Style

"Red-beans-and-rice" is all one word in New Orleans. City ordinance requires that red beans always be served with rice and hot sauce. Who needs anything else?

½ pound dried red beans
1 large onion, finely chopped
1 red bell pepper, finely chopped
2 stalks celery, finely chopped
1 can (14.5-ounce) of diced tomatoes
3 large garlic cloves, pressed
1 tablespoon olive oil
1 teaspoon cumin
½ teaspoon cinnamon
¼ teaspoon cayenne

1. Soak the beans in water overnight.
2. Cover the beans with at least 1 inch of water and simmer covered for 1 ½ hours. Add water to prevent the beans from drying.
3. Sweat the onion, garlic, and spices in olive oil for 10 minutes. Add the red bell pepper, celery, and spices, and sauté for another 10 minutes.
4. Add the beans, water, and spices. Cover and simmer for 1 ½ hours. Add water to prevent the beans from drying.

Serves 4
150 calories per serving, 2.7 g total fat (17 percent of calories), 0.4 g saturated, 1.7 g monounsaturated, 0.3 g polyunsaturated, 0 cholesterol, 150 mg sodium, 6.7 g fiber

## Boston Baked Beans

A regular molasses and rum trade between Boston and Jamaica in colonial America launched this New England tradition. Sue gave our fifteen-month-old grandson a full plate, which he immediately downed, and then cried when she wouldn't give him any more. She said that little guys need variety. What a mean grandmother!

1 pound dry Great Northern beans
1 onion, chopped
2 garlic cloves, pressed
1 piece ginger root (2 inches), peeled and chopped
¼ cup molasses
¼ cup ketchup
¼ cup mustard
1 teaspoon *herbes de Provence*
1 bay leaf
1 cup herb-seasoned bread stuffing

1. Soak the beans overnight and decant the water. Boil them in 2 quarts of water, and decant most of the liquid, saving some to add to the beans during baking if necessary.
2. Add the onion, garlic, ginger root, *herbes de Provence,* bay leaf, molasses, ketchup, and mustard. Sweating the onion and garlic is not necessary because of the long baking time.
3. Add enough of the saved liquid to cover the beans, and bake in a covered casserole dish at 300° F for 4 to 6 hours. Check occasionally to be sure that the beans don't become too dry; add water if necessary.
4. Remove the cover ½ hour from the end of baking and sprinkle the bread stuffing on the beans. Leave uncovered for the rest of the baking.

Serves 12
140 calories per serving, 0.4 g total fat (3 percent of calories), 0 g saturated, 0 g monounsaturated, 0.1 g polyunsaturated, 0 mg cholesterol, 6.0 g fiber, 150 mg sodium

## Cannellini Beans and Mushrooms

This hardy vegetable dish can serve as a main course in a completely vegetarian meal, but it also works well garnished with broiled chicken. One serving has only 140 calories, so have two.

½ pound dried cannellini or Great Northern beans
1 pound mushrooms cut into large bite-sized pieces
½ onion, chopped
1 garlic cloves, chopped
4 stems Italian parsley, reserve the leaves
2 sprigs thyme
½ teaspoon ground black pepper
1 bay leaf
1 tablespoon olive oil
1 Meyer lemon for juice
4 cups water

1. Soak beans in water overnight and decant the water.
2. Make a bouquet garni with the parsley stems, fresh thyme, and bay leaf tied together with a string.
3. Sweat the onion and garlic in a large sauce pot for about 10 minutes. Add the beans and the bouquet garni to 4 cups of water. Simmer for 1 ½ hours. Add more water if needed.
4. Remove and the bouquet garni, but reserve the liquid.
5. In a skillet, brown the mushrooms in a small amount of olive oil until they stop giving off liquid. Add the lemon juice and pepper and heat until the pan is almost dry.
6. Combine the beans, mushrooms, and ¼ cup of the reserved liquid and cook until well combined and hot.
7. Stir in the chopped parsley leaves and serve.

Serves 6
140 calories per serving, 2.7 g total fat (18 percent of calories), 0.4 g saturated, 1.7 g monounsaturated, 0.3 g polyunsaturated, 0 mg cholesterol, 2 mg sodium, 6.0 g fiber

## Cauliflower in a Spicy Tomato Sauce

Many different savory spices work with cauliflower, which may serve as a main course garnished with a small broiled chicken breast or nonfat chicken-apple sausage as described in the Tips and Tricks section. The spices selected here blend Mediterranean and South Asian flavors. Brown rice or wheat berry pilaf and a green salad complete the meal.

1 head cauliflower
1 can (14.5-ounce) diced tomatoes
½ small can tomato paste
¾ cup chicken stock
½ onion, chopped
1 tablespoon olive oil
1 tablespoon curry powder
1 teaspoon sugar
¼ cup chopped cilantro (Chinese parsley)

1. Cut the florets into about 24 pieces and brown in ½ tablespoon of olive oil for about 3 or 4 minutes.
2. Remove and sweat the onions on low for 10 minutes in another ½ tablespoon of olive oil adding the curry powder and sugar.
3. Add the diced tomatoes, tomato paste, and the cauliflower florets, plus some chicken stock to thin the tomato sauce as desired. Cover and simmer for about 20 minutes until the cauliflower is tender.
4. Sprinkle with cilantro and serve.

Serves 6
80 calories per serving, 4.5 g fat (35 percent of calories), 0.6 g saturated fat, 2.7 g monounsaturated, 0.6 g polyunsaturated, 0 mg cholesterol, 300 mg sodium, 1.6 g fiber

## Cauliflower with Herbed Crumb Topping

Bread crumbs, garlic, and olive oil dress up a simple vegetable dish.

1 head cauliflower
1½ slices of crusty whole grain bread crumbed (see Tips and Tricks)
1 tablespoon olive oil
2 cloves garlic, pressed
¼ teaspoon black pepper
2 green onions, sliced
4 or 5 sprigs of parsley, chopped

1. Cut the florets into about 24 pieces and steam in a covered pot for about 8 to 10 minutes.
2. Drain and spread the florets in a baking dish.
3. Mix the green onions, parsley, oil, and garlic with the bread crumbs in a plastic bag, and sprinkle over the cauliflower.
4. Bake at 425°F uncovered for 10 minutes.

Serves 6
64 calories per serving, 2.0 g fat (26 percent of calories), 0.3 g saturated fat, 1.2 g monounsaturated, 0.3 g polyunsaturated, 0 mg cholesterol, 215 mg sodium, 1.7 g fiber

## Dutch Mash

Dutch mash is a winter holiday substitution for ordinary mashed potatoes. The mixed root vegetables, combined with apples, onions, and nutmeg, give it a hint of sweetness that complements the roast turkey or chicken for a Thanksgiving or Christmas dinner. A neighbor from Sue's childhood had brought the recipe for Dutch mash back from Holland after the Second World War. At that time, ham was only for export, so the Dutch invented this delicious vegetarian alternative. Ham is plentiful in Holland now, but Dutch mash is still popular.

5 boiling potatoes, scrubbed and quartered
4 carrots cut into 1-inch pieces
1 rutabaga in 1-inch pieces
3 apples, peeled, cored, and quartered
1 onion peeled and quartered
1 cup dried milk powder
1 cup cold chicken stock
¼ teaspoon nutmeg
¼ teaspoon ground black pepper

1. Boil the vegetables and apple until soft, about 30 minutes. Drain.
2. Return the vegetables and apple to the pot and mash. In a separate bowl, whisk the milk powder and spices into the cold chicken stock.
3. Gradually add enough chicken stock to bring the mashed vegetables to the desired consistency.
4. Warm and serve.

Serves 8
140 calories per serving, 0.3 g fat (1 percent of calories), 0 g saturated fat, 0.1 g monounsaturated, 0.1 g polyunsaturated, 0 mg cholesterol, 200 mg sodium, 4 g fiber

## Mashed Potatoes and Carrots

This recipe is a quick and easy variation of Dutch mash. Carrots and garlic elevate ordinary powdered mashed potatoes and give them a sweet flavor.

1 packet of powdered mashed potatoes
3 carrots in 2-inch chunks
3 cloves of garlic, pressed
½ onion, finely chopped
1 tablespoon olive oil
¾ cup powdered skim milk
2⅔ cups boiling chicken stock
1 teaspoon thyme
¼ teaspoon black pepper
4 or 5 sprigs parsley, chopped

1. Boil carrots in water until soft. Purée in a food processor.
2. Sweat the onions and garlic on low for 10 minutes.
3. Add the 2 ⅔ cups boiling chicken stock and briskly stir in the powdered milk and dry mashed potatoes using a whisk.
4. Whip together with the puréed carrots and black pepper.
5. Garnish with the parsley.

Serves 6
130 calories per serving, 2.2 g fat (14 percent of calories), 0.3 g saturated fat, 1.5 g monounsaturated, 0.4 g polyunsaturated, 6 mg cholesterol, 200 mg sodium, 1.6 g fiber

## Roasted New Potatoes

Add other vegetables, such as carrots, rutabaga, butternut squash, or sweet potatoes in large chunks.

20 small new potatoes
1 tablespoon olive oil
1 clove garlic, pressed
4 to 5 sprigs rosemary

1. Cut the potatoes in half and put them into a plastic sack with the olive oil, garlic, and rosemary. Shake to coat the potatoes and place them on a baking sheet.
2. Bake for 1 ½ hours at 350° F, turning once.

Serves 6
225 calories per serving, 3.6 g fat (15 percent of calories), 0.4 g saturated fat, 2.5 g monounsaturated, 0.7g polyunsaturated, 0 mg cholesterol, 80 mg sodium, 3.0 g fiber

## Savory Baked Apples

The words savory and apples seem a contradiction, but these apples baked with rosemary and onions are wonderful. Try it with broiled marinated chicken or sautéed sablefish and a baked sweet potato.

4 apples, cored and peeled into 1-inch chunks
1 onion, coarsely chopped
1 tablespoon olive oil
1 teaspoon rosemary or one 5-inch piece of fresh rosemary
½ pound nonfat chicken sausage (see Tips and Tricks)

1. Fry the onions and sausage on medium low for 10 minutes.
2. Place in a covered baking dish together with the apples and rose-mary and bake at 400° F for 30 minutes. Uncover and bake for an additional 15 minutes.
3. Serve with a baked sweet potato or other vegetable.

Serves 4
175 calories per serving, 4.0 g total fat (20 percent of calories), 0.5 g saturated, 2.6 g monounsaturated, 0.5 g polyunsaturated, 1 mg cholesterol, 100 mg sodium, 4.2 g fiber

# *Bread*

Sue has baked each of these breads for many years. A powerful mixer with a dough hook simplifies the preparation of the dough, so that homemade bread can become an everyday treat. Commercially sold bread contains significant amounts of sodium, usually between one hundred and two hundred milligrams per slice. None of the following recipes includes salt, and none is required, but you may add a small amount if you feel so compelled. Keep in mind that one teaspoon of salt equals sixteen hundred milligrams of sodium. Divided among twenty slices, that's only about two hundred milligrams of salt and eighty milligrams of sodium per slice. However, if you are trying to keep sodium intake below three thousand milligrams per day, consider omitting, or at least reducing, the amount of salt added to the dough.

## Dark Chocolate Rye

This spectacular dark bread always disappears rapidly. A small quantity of cocoa gives it a cake-like taste that complements many of the hardy dishes in the previous sections.

2 cups rye flour
3¾ cups flour, half white and half whole-wheat
¼ cup cocoa
1 package of dry yeast
½ cup molasses
1 tablespoon vegetable oil (not olive oil)
1½ cups lukewarm water

1. Place yeast in a bowl with the water, molasses, vegetable oil, and 1 cup of flour and mix using dough hook. Let stand for 15 minutes to assure that the yeast is active, indicated by tiny bubbles in the dough.
2. Add the rest of the ingredients, except for 1 cup of flour to add gradually until the dough forms a firm ball around the dough hook.
3. Cover with a towel and let the dough rise in the mixing bowl for about 1 hour or until double.
4. Punch down and form into a loaf on a greased cookie sheet coated with a thin layer of cornmeal.
5. Cover with a towel and let rise for another hour.
6. Bake at 375° F for 35 to 40 minutes.

Makes about 20 slices
140 calories per slice, 1.3 g total fat (8 percent of total), 0.2 g saturated, 0.2 g monounsaturated, 0.4 g polyunsaturated, 0 mg cholesterol, 3 mg sodium, 3.4 g fiber

## Crusty Whole Wheat Walnut Bread

San Francisco bakers use hot ovens with steam jets for making crusty sourdough bread, turning off the steam to create the crust during the last few minutes of baking. Most of us don't have a special bread oven, but by placing the dough in a Dutch oven, the enclosed space captures steam from the wet dough to mimic the effect. For the last 10 or 15 minutes of baking, remove the lid of the Dutch oven to allow the crust to form.

Some French bakers recommend using a smaller amount of yeast than usual and allowing the dough to rise slowly overnight for 18 hours to enrich the flavor of the bread. For the second rising, place the dough on a large piece of lightly-oiled parchment paper laid across a round pan, such as a frying pan with a diameter slightly smaller than the Dutch oven's. You will be able to use the parchment paper to transfer the dough to the Dutch oven more easily before baking, as well as for removing the bread later from the hot Dutch oven.

3 cups of flour, half and half white and whole wheat
1 cup walnuts toasted for 10 minutes at 350° F
¼ teaspoon of yeast
(Optional: 1 teaspoon salt optional)
7 ounces of lukewarm water
3 ounces of red wine
1 tablespoon vinegar

1. Mix the flour, yeast, walnuts, and salt in a mixing bowl, and add the lukewarm water, red wine, and vinegar. Turn on the mixer to combine all of the ingredients and then form the dough into a ball. Cover and allow it to rise overnight.
2. Knead the dough for 2 or 3 minutes. Place the dough on a large piece of oiled parchment paper laid across a 10-inch frying pan and allow it to rise another 2 hours.
3. Preheat the empty Dutch oven to 500° F. in the main oven.
4. Cut 1 or 2 slits on the top of the dough and transfer it into the hot Dutch oven using the edges of the parchment paper as handles. Cover the Dutch oven and bake the bread at 425° F for 30 minutes.
5. Remove the Dutch oven lid and bake 10 minutes longer to form the crust.
6 Transfer the bread from the Dutch oven to a cooling rack using the parchment paper edges again, and allow it to cool for 1 to 2 hours.

Makes about 14 slices
155 calories per slice, 6.0 g total fat (35 percent of total), 0.6 g saturated, 3.5 g monounsaturated, 1.9 g polyunsaturated, 0 mg cholesterol, 75 mg sodium, 2.5 g fiber

## Oatmeal Bread

Serve the oatmeal bread with soup, salad, or any main course, but it is especially good toasted for breakfast.

1 cup rolled oatmeal
1 cup of whole wheat flour
3 cups of unbleached white flour
¼ cup honey or molasses
1½ cups water
1 package of yeast
1 tablespoon canola, corn, or safflower oil

1. Warm the water to approximately 100° F and stir in the yeast.
2. Combine all of the ingredients in a mixing bowl and knead with the dough hook. If needed, add more flour or water to make a firm batter.
3. Cover with a towel and let rise until double in about 45 minutes.
4. Shape into a loaf and place into a greased bread pan to rise again for about 45 minutes more.
5. Bake at 375° F for about 35 to 40 minutes.

Makes about 20 slices
100 calories per slice, 1.0 g total fat (10 percent of total), 0.1 g saturated, 0.3 g monounsaturated, 0.5 g polyunsaturated, 0 mg cholesterol, 3 mg sodium, 1.4 g fiber

## Onion Cottage Cheese Bread

This recipe came from Sue's friend Kathryn Langston, whose mother was baking both onion cottage cheese bread and shredded wheat bread back in the 1930s. Sue modified them by blending white and whole wheat flour.

5 cups flour, half white and half whole wheat
2 cups lukewarm cottage cheese
4 teaspoons sugar
2 tablespoons onion, finely chopped
2 tablespoons vegetable oil
4 teaspoons caraway seeds
½ teaspoon baking soda
¼ cup egg substitute

1. Mix all the ingredients beginning with 3 cups of flour and adding the last 2 cups gradually to make a firm dough.
2. Let rise until double. Punch down and place into a greased round casserole dishes.
3. Let rise again for about 40 minutes and bake at 350° F for 40 to 45 minutes.

Makes about 20 slices
135 calories per slice, 1.7 g total fat (11 percent of calories), 0.1 g saturated, 0.3 g monounsaturated, 0.5 g polyunsaturated, 0 mg cholesterol, 65 mg sodium, 1.4 g fiber

## Shredded Wheat Bread

A few years ago, every grandchild had a grandmother who made shredded wheat bread just like this.

2 large shredded wheat biscuits, or 2 cups of bite-sized biscuits
1 cup whole wheat flour
3½ cups of white flour
1½ cups boiling water
1 teaspoon vegetable oil
¼ cup honey and molasses mixed
1 package of yeast

1. Pour boiling water over shredded wheat biscuits. Add oil, honey, and molasses, and let the mix cool to lukewarm.
2. Add yeast and flour by cupfuls to make a firm batter and knead with dough hook.
3. Cover with a towel and let rise until double. Shape into a loaf and place into greased bread pan. Let rise again for about 30 to 40 minutes.
4. Bake at 375° F for 40 minutes.

Makes about 20 slices
100 calories per slice, 1.0 g total fat (7 percent of total), 0.1 g saturated, 0.2 monounsaturated, 0.4 g polyunsaturated, 0 mg cholesterol, 3 mg sodium, 0.9 g fiber

## Cornbread

Cornbread complements any bean dish, but especially Mexican turkey chili mole in the poultry section. It has saved us when unexpected guests arrive, and we're out of bread. Nobody has ever complained about piping-hot cornbread as a substitute for anything store-bought.

1 cup corn meal
1 cup flour
1 tablespoon brown sugar
2 teaspoons baking powder
¼ cup egg substitute
¼ cup olive oil
½ cup nonfat milk (may use powdered milk)
(Optional: ½ cup frozen corn)
(Optional: ¼ cup chopped red bell pepper)
(Optional: ¼ cup sunflower seeds)

1. Mix and place in a greased baking pan.
2. Bake at 400° F for 20 minutes.

Serves 8
140 calories per serving, 2.5 g total fat (16 percent of calories), 0.3 g saturated, 1.5 g monounsaturated, 0.5 g polyunsaturated, 0 mg cholesterol, 25 mg sodium, 2.0 g fiber

## Patty Cakes

Patty cakes are whole grain biscuits with sunflower seeds, and they are very filling. When Sue makes them, our grandchildren say: "That's pretty crunchy, Grandma." Their word "crunchy" refers to the granola that they associate with the hippy culture from which patty cakes emerged.

2 cups unbleached white flour
1 cup rolled oats
1 cup whole wheat flour
½ cup toasted sunflower seeds
1 cup nonfat milk
¼ cup Canola oil
¼ black pepper
2 teaspoons baking powder

1. Combine the dry ingredients in a bowl.
2. Gradually mix in the milk and oil.
3. Shape the patty cakes with your hands and place on a cookie sheet lined with parchment paper.
4. Bake in an oven preheated to 400° F for 20 minutes.

Makes 12 biscuits
160 calories per biscuit, 5.0 g total fat (24 percent of total), 0.4 g saturated, 2.2 g monounsaturated, 2.3 g polyunsaturated, 0 mg cholesterol, 200 mg sodium, 2.1 g fiber

## Whole Grain Blueberry Biscuits

Our daughter Sarah won a prize for her recipe for blueberry biscuits in *Better Homes and Gardens,* March 2006. Sue modified her own version to fit the Nutritional Guidelines for Americans and doubled the quantities to fit the appetites of eight hungry grandchildren.

1 cup white flour
1 cup whole wheat flour
½ cup oatmeal
4 tablespoons whole bran cereal
1 cup of fresh blueberries
½ cup powdered nonfat milk in 1 ¼ cups water
3 tablespoons of canola oil
2 teaspoons sugar
2 teaspoons baking powder

1. Combine all the ingredients except for the blueberries into a mixing bowl and stir.
2. Gently stir in the blueberries.
3. Drop the batter onto a lightly greased cookie sheet to make about 12 biscuits.
4. Bake at 400° F for about 20 minutes, or until browned.

Makes 12 biscuits
145 calories per biscuit, 4.2 g total fat (26 percent of total), 0.4 g saturated, 2.2 g monounsaturated, 1.2 g polyunsaturated, 0 mg cholesterol, 120 mg sodium, 2.5 g fiber

## Popovers

Popovers are very light, puffy, hollow muffins that rise over the rim of the baking tin. British chefs make them using the fat from roast beef and name them Yorkshire pudding. Our recipe is easy to prepare and much lower in calories than the English version, so popovers don't have to wait for special occasions. Sue serves them with many of the soup, salad, and poultry recipes in the book.

1 cup flour, half unbleached white and half whole wheat
½ cup egg substitute
1 cup nonfat milk, or ⅓ cup powdered nonfat milk in 1 cup water
½ teaspoon black pepper
¼ teaspoon nutmeg

1. Add the dry ingredients to the milk and egg substitute, and mix well with a spoon.
2. Lightly grease a muffin tin with a polyunsaturated vegetable oil and fill each cup ⅔ full with the batter.
3. Place the tin in a cold oven and turn on the heat to 450° F. Bake for 25 minutes. Don't peek or the muffins may collapse.

Makes 12 muffins
45 calories per muffin, 0.2 g total fat (4 percent of calories), 0 g saturated, 0 g monounsaturated, 1 g polyunsaturated, 0 cholesterol, 0.8 g fiber, 10 mg sodium

# *Salads*

## Four Salad Dressings

Make the following dressings in a jar and keep in the refrigerator for up to 10 days. Each serving is one tablespoon.

Mustard Vinaigrette
- 2 tablespoon mustard
- ¼ cup red wine vinegar or cider vinegar
- ¼ cup olive oil

Garlic Dressing
- 1 clove garlic crushed
- 1 teaspoon mustard
- ½ cup red wine vinegar
- ¼ cup olive oil
- ¼ cup canola oil
- ½ teaspoon ketchup

Lemon Vinaigrette
- 2 lemons for juice
- ¼ cup olive oil
- ¼ cup canola oil
- 1 teaspoon mustard
- 2 teaspoons paprika

Jam Vinaigrette (Add ingredients to a jam jar with remnants, heat in a microwave for 30 seconds, and shake.)
- ¼ cup balsamic vinegar
- ¼ cup distilled white vinegar
- ½ cup olive oil
- 1 teaspoon mustard

All dressings are about 70 calories per tablespoon, 7.0 g total fat (96 percent of calories), 0.9 g saturated, 5.2 g monounsaturated, 1.9 g polyunsaturated, 0 cholesterol, 0 sodium, 0 fiber

## Salade Niçoise

Summer in Provence and California have much in common reflected in this variation of *salade Niçoise* with avocado. Serve it with a loaf of crunchy multigrain bread. It's perfect for a warm evening on the terrace with a glass of iced tea.

6 tuna steaks, ahi or tombo, about 4 ounces each
4 ounces fresh French string beans
2 tomatoes in sections
6 large lettuce leaves
1 small shallot, peeled and chopped
1 small avocado in ¾-inch pieces
1 tablespoon olive oil
1 tablespoon wine vinegar
1 tablespoon chopped tarragon
1 tablespoon black peppercorns, crushed
1 tablespoon *herbes de Provence* (thyme, savory, marjoram, oregano)
¼ teaspoon ground black pepper

1. Steam the string beans for 3 minutes, but no longer, and then plunge into cold water to stop the cooking. Drain.
2. Mix the vinegar, shallots, tarragon, pepper, and olive oil in a large salad bowl. Fold in the tomatoes and avocado gently.
3. Wash, dry, and tear the lettuce into smaller leaves. Add to the salad bowl, and toss.
4. Pat the crushed pepper and herbs de Provence into the tuna and sprinkle with olive oil. Sear the tuna on high in a large skillet, or broil, but no more than 2 minutes on a side.
5. Serve the tuna on top of the salad.

Serves 6
350 calories per serving, 21 g fat (54 percent of calories), 3.1 g saturated, 13.4 g monounsaturated, 2.3 g polyunsaturated, 47 mg cholesterol, 50 mg sodium, 5.7 g fiber

Variation
Add cubed boiled new potatoes marinated in olive oil, wine vinegar, and capers. The French often add a hard-boiled egg too.

## Shrimp Salad

We usually put shrimp salad on the menu for family gatherings and parties, especially in the summer. However, we have four children and eight grandchildren, so we triple the recipe. Serve it with iced tea and multigrain bread, or include it in a buffet.

1 pound small cooked shrimp
3 stalks and leaves celery, sliced
2 tablespoons capers, rinsed
2 green onions sliced, or ½ red onion, diced

Dressing:
  1 clove garlic, pressed
  1 teaspoon Dijon mustard
  2 Meyer lemons for juice
  1½ tablespoon olive oil
  ½ teaspoon fresh ground black pepper

1. Make a salad dressing in the bottom of a bowl by whisking together the last five ingredients.
2. Carefully mix in the shrimp, celery, capers, and green onions taking care not to break apart the shrimp.
3. Let the salad sit in the refrigerator for at least one hour to help blend the flavors.
4. Serve over lettuce with sliced fresh tomatoes.

Serves 4
175 calories per serving, 7.2 g fat (38 percent of calories), 1.1 g saturated, 4.1 g monounsaturated, 1.2 g polyunsaturated, 25 mg cholesterol, 200 mg sodium, 0.5 g fiber

## Mixed Greens with Vinaigrette, Feta Cheese, Walnuts, and Cranberries

The Woodside Bakery near Stanford has served a salad like this for many years as a main course for lunch on the terrace. It's still the most popular item on the menu.
Mixed greens for four, washed and torn

½ cup walnuts
½ cup dried cranberries or cherries
4 ounces nonfat feta cheese
Dressing:
  2 tablespoons white wine vinegar
  1 tablespoon Dijon mustard
  2 tablespoons olive oil

1. Roast the walnuts in an oven at 320° F for 20 minutes.
2. Combine and whisk the vinegar and mustard. Slowly add the olive oil, while whisking constantly.
3. Toss the greens with the dressing.
4. Top each salad with the feta cheese, cranberries, and walnuts.

Serves 4
270 calories per serving, 23 g total fat (77 percent of calories), 1.9 g saturated, 8.8 g monounsaturated, 11.4 g polyunsaturated, 0 cholesterol, 260 mg sodium, 2.5 g fiber

## Tomato, Cucumber, and Bell Pepper Salad

This salad is the perfect complement to Mediterranean and Californian cuisine where the long warm months deliver an abundant supply of sweet red tomatoes.

1 head green leaf lettuce, washed
4 ripe tomatoes, sliced
1 long thin-skinned cucumber, sliced
2 green bell peppers, sliced
Dressing:
  2 tablespoons olive oil
  2 tablespoons red wine vinegar
  ½ teaspoon ketchup
  1 garlic clove pressed
  ¼ teaspoon paprika
  ⅛ teaspoon black pepper

1. Line a chilled platter with the washed lettuce and arrange overlapping slices of tomato, cucumber, and bell peppers.
2. Pour the dressing just before serving.

Serves 4
90 calories per serving, 7.4 g total fat (74 percent of calories), 1.0 g saturated, 5.2 g monounsaturated, 0.8 g polyunsaturated, 0 cholesterol, 3 mg sodium, 1.3 g fiber

# *Appendix: Dietary Guidelines Advisory Committee Membership 2005*

**Chair**

Janet King, PhD, RD
Children's Hospital Oakland Research Institute and
University of California Davis and Berkeley
Oakland, California

**Members**

Lawrence Appel, MD, MPH
Johns Hopkins University
School of Medicine
Baltimore, Maryland

Yvonne Bronner, ScD, RD, LD
Morgan State University
Baltimore, Maryland

Benjamin Caballero, MD, PhD
Johns Hopkins University
Bloomberg School of Public Health
and School of Medicine
Baltimore, Maryland

Carlos Camargo, MD, DrPH
Harvard University
Boston, Massachusetts

Fergus Clydesdale, PhD
University of Massachusetts,
Amherst
Amherst, Massachusetts

Penny Kris-Etherton, PhD, RD
Pennsylvania State University
University Park, Pennsylvania

Joanne Lupton, PhD
Texas A&M University
College Station, Texas

Theresa Nicklas, Dr. PH, MPH, LDN
Children's Nutrition Research
Center
Baylor College of Medicine
Houston, Texas

Russell Pate, PhD
University of South Carolina
Columbia, South Carolina

F. Xavier Pi-Sunyer, MD, MPH
St. Luke's-Roosevelt Hospital
Center and Columbia University
New York, New York

Vay Liang W. Go, MD
David Geffen School of Medicine
University of California at Los Angeles
Los Angeles, California

Connie Weaver, PhD
Purdue University
West Lafayette, Indiana

# *What are Triglycerides, Saturated Fat, Unsaturated Fat, Trans Fat, LDL, VLDL, and HDL?*

The terms saturated, unsaturated, and trans fat all refer to types of triglycerides, which constitute more than 99 percent of fat in the diet. Dietary triglycerides clear from the bloodstream within a few hours after eating, but the liver can make triglycerides by transforming glucose (sugar), a process that continues even while fasting. The body converts all ingested simple or complex carbohydrates and any excess protein above the daily requirements into glucose, which we can either use immediately or store as glycogen in tissues. Glycogen can rapidly transform back to glucose as the main source of energy in the fasting state to maintain the blood sugar in a normal range. Even during fasting, the liver still converts some glucose to triglycerides, but normally only in very small amounts.

The terms LDL (low density lipoprotein), VLDL (very low density lipoprotein), and HDL (high density lipoprotein) refer to blood-borne lipoproteins that transport fat.

- VLDL transports triglyceride made by the liver to fat cells for storage. A moderate risk of cardiovascular disease accompanies abnormally high fasting VLDL levels.
- LDL is the main transport vehicle for cholesterol in the bloodstream; abnormally high levels indicate a high risk for cardiovascular disease. Cholesterol amounts to less than one percent of dietary fat, but even small increases in LDL can lead to atherosclerosis.
- HDL is protective against the formation of atherosclerosis, presumably because it absorbs cholesterol and triglycerides. High levels of HDL indicate a low risk of cardiovascular disease.

Triglycerides contain three fatty acid chains. All the carbon atom sites are saturated with hydrogen atoms on the fatty acid chains of saturated fats, while unsaturated means that some sites remain available. With unsaturated fatty acids, two adjacent unsaturated carbon atoms share a double bond instead of the more usual single bond. Most dietary fatty acids have chains containing either sixteen or eighteen carbon atoms. Omega-3 and omega-6 fatty acids refer to those found in specific types of unsaturated fats; the numbers indicate the position of the double bond on the chain, which is usually longer than the typical fatty acid chain that has sixteen or eighteen carbon atoms (Stryer 1981, 226–227).

Saturated

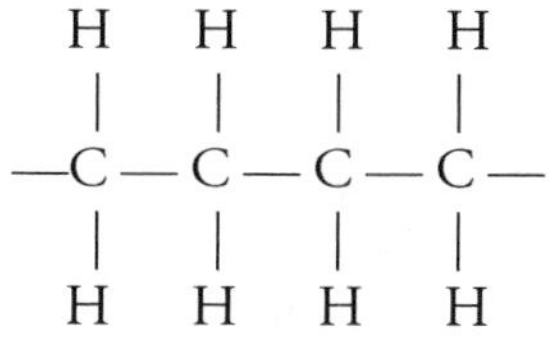

```
  H   H   H   H
  |   |   |   |
—C — C — C — C —
  |   |   |   |
  H   H   H   H
```

Unsaturated

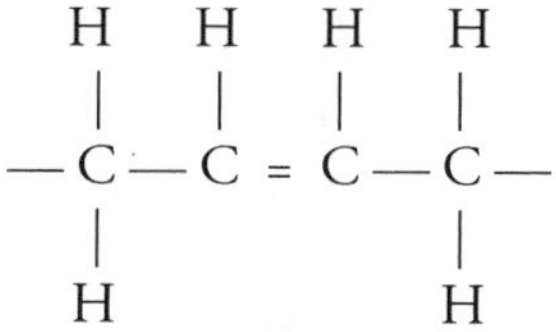

```
  H   H   H   H
  |   |   |   |
—C — C = C — C —
  |           |
  H           H
```

Monounsaturated means that one site in the fatty chain has a double bond, while polyunsaturated means there are two or three double bonds in the chain. The process called "partial hydrogenation" converts double bonds to single bonds by adding hydrogen atoms at the sites of double bonds to form trans fat. In the process, a vegetable oil becomes more solid, such as with stick margarine or the fat typically used in deep frying. Saturated fatty acid chains are usually straighter, called the trans conformation, which is more compact, and consequently, more solid at room temperature. They also have a longer shelf life than unsaturated fats and do not give off smoke at high temperatures like unsaturated fats. Where double bonds exist, a chain forms a sharp angle, called the cis conformation, so that mono- or polyunsaturated fatty acids form twists and kinks (cis) that make them more loosely packed, and thus unsaturated fats are liquid at room temperature, but smoky when they are heated to high temperature (Mozaffarian 2006, 1601-13).

Fat is inefficient as an energy source, whether from the diet or produced in the liver. Our minimum daily requirements for dietary fats are very small, because the liver can make most of the fat we need by transforming either carbohydrate or protein into fat. However, all of us require very small amounts of essential fatty acids that the liver is incapable of making. Essential fatty acids all come from fish or vegetable sources; there are no essential saturated fatty acids. Foods containing saturated fat, whether naturally or from partial hydrogenation, have no necessary nutrition value. Consequently, the fats in red meat, dairy fat, cocoa butter, or trans fat are empty calories.

Fat metabolism is slow and generates byproducts like ketoacids that require glucose and insulin to eliminate, but fat allows concentration and storage of huge amounts of energy with minimum space in fat cells. Our capacity to store energy as fat is almost unlimited as evidenced by observing obese people. On the other hand, stored carbohydrate in the form of glycogen requires a substantial amount of water, consuming a large amount of space and adding weight. In the fasting state, we always use the conversion of glycogen to glucose as the preferred source of energy, but glycogen stores last only about four to twelve hours, depending upon the amount of physical activity. Athletes who use up all of their glycogen stores "bonk" or "hit the wall;" their high energy demands exceed their immediate supply, because fat metabolism is too slow and generates large amounts of lactic acid that impairs muscular activity. Serious athletes in training typically restrict fat intake and consume most of their calories in the form of carbohydrate to maximize glycogen stores and improve endurance.

Most people should restrict fat intake to no more than 25 to 30 percent of total calories, but should assure consumption of adequate amounts of essential fatty acids from vegetable or fish sources. Anyone with abnormal lipoproteins should completely abstain from foods high in saturated fat or trans fat.

# *Food Values of Common Portions*

| | *calories* | *total fat g* | *% of calories* | *saturated g* | *monounsatt g* | *polyunsat g* | *cholesterol mg* | *fiber g* | *sodium mg* |
|---|---|---|---|---|---|---|---|---|---|
| **Grains** | | | | | | | | | |
| barley, ¼ cup dry | 180 | 0 | 0% | 0 | 0 | 0 | 0 | 8.0 | 0 |
| capellini, ⅔ cup dry | 204 | 1.3 | 6% | 0.3 | 0.2 | 0.8 | 0 | 1.9 | 3 |
| cereal, cooked, multigrain, ⅓ cup | 160 | 3 | 17% | 0.5 | | | 0 | 6.0 | 0 |
| cornmeal, 1 cup dry | 442 | 4.4 | 9% | 0.6 | 1.2 | 2.0 | 0 | 8.9 | 43 |
| couscous, cooked, 1 cup | 200 | 0.3 | 1% | 0.1 | 0 | 0.1 | 0 | 2.5 | 9 |
| couscous, whole grain, ⅓ cup dry | 210 | 1 | 1% | 0.1 | 0 | 0.1 | 0 | 5.0 | 0 |
| flour, white, 1 cup | 455 | 1.2 | 2% | 0.2 | 0.1 | 0.5 | 0 | 3.4 | 3 |
| flour, whole wheat, 1 cup | 407 | 2.2 | 5% | 0.4 | 0.3 | 0.9 | 0 | 14.6 | 6 |
| flour, rye, 1 cup | 415 | 3.4 | 7% | 0.4 | 0.4 | 1.5 | 0 | 28.9 | 2 |
| noodles, egg white, 1 ¾ cup dry | 196 | 1.2 | 6% | 0.3 | 0.2 | 0.8 | 0 | 1.8 | 13 |
| macaroni, 1 cup cooked | 197 | 0.9 | 4% | 0.1 | 0.1 | 0.4 | 0 | 1.8 | 1 |
| oatmeal, rolled, ½ cup dry | 140 | 2.5 | 16% | 0.5 | 1.0 | 1.0 | 0 | 4.0 | 0 |
| oatmeal, steel cut, ¼ cup dry | 150 | 2.5 | 15% | 0.5 | 1.0 | 1.0 | 0 | 4.0 | 0 |
| polenta, ½ cup dry | 125 | 0.5 | 0.4% | 0 | 0.2 | 0.2 | 0 | 0.5 | 0 |
| rice, white, 1 cup cooked | 205 | 0.4 | 2% | 0.1 | 0.1 | 0.1 | 0 | 0.6 | 2 |
| rice, brown, 1 cup cooked | 180 | 1.5 | 8% | 0.3 | 0.5 | 0.5 | 0 | 3.5 | 10 |
| spaghetti, 1 cup cooked, 2 oz | 197 | 0.9 | 4% | 0.1 | 0.1 | 0.4 | 0 | 2.4 | 1 |

| | *calories* | *total fat g* | *% of calories* | *saturated g* | *monounsatt g* | *polyunsat g* | *cholesterol mg* | *fiber g* | *sodium mg* |
|---|---|---|---|---|---|---|---|---|---|
| spaghetti, whole wheat, dry ⅛ lb | 187 | 1 | 5% | 0 | 0 | 0 | 0 | 4.0 | 1 |
| **Vegetables** | | | | | | | | | |
| asparagus ½ cup, 6 spears | 22 | 0.3 | 12% | 0.1 | 0.0 | 0.1 | 0 | 1.4 | 10 |
| avocado, raw, 1 medium | 306 | 30 | 88% | 4.5 | 19.4 | 3.5 | 0 | 8.5 | 21 |
| beans, great northern, 1 cup boiled | 209 | 0.8 | 3% | 0.2 | 0.0 | 0.3 | 0 | 12.4 | 4 |
| beans, black, 1 cup boiled | 227 | 0.9 | 4% | 0.2 | 0.1 | 0.4 | 0 | 15.0 | 2 |
| green beans, ½ cup boiled | 22 | 0.2 | 8% | 0.0 | 0.0 | 0.1 | 0 | 2.0 | 2 |
| beans, kidney, 1 cup boiled | 225 | 0.9 | 4% | 0.1 | 0.1 | 0.5 | 0 | 13.1 | 4 |
| beans, lima, boiled, 1 cup | 216 | 0.7 | 3% | 0.2 | 0.1 | 0.3 | 0 | 13.2 | 4 |
| broccoli, ½ cup raw | 22 | 0.3 | 12% | 0.0 | 0.0 | 0.1 | 0 | 2.3 | 20 |
| cabbage, ½ cup raw shredded | 2 | 0 | 0% | 0.0 | 0.0 | 0.0 | 0 | 0.8 | 6 |
| carrots, 1 med raw | 31 | 0.1 | 3% | 0.0 | 0.0 | 0.1 | 0 | 2.2 | 25 |
| cauliflower, ½ cup boiled | 14 | 0.3 | 19% | 0.0 | 0.0 | 0.1 | 0 | 1.7 | 9 |
| celery 1 stalk | 6 | 0.1 | 15% | 0.0 | 0.0 | 0.0 | 0 | 0.7 | 35 |
| chickpeas, 1 cup boiled | 269 | 4.2 | 14% | 0.4 | 1.0 | 1.9 | 0 | 12.5 | 11 |
| corn, ½ cup boiled | 89 | 1 | 10% | 0.2 | 0.3 | 0.5 | 0 | 2.3 | 14 |
| garlic 3 cloves | 13 | 0 | 0% | 0.0 | 0.0 | 0.0 | 0 | 0.2 | 2 |
| leeks, ½ cup boiled | 8 | 0.1 | 11% | 0.0 | 0.0 | 0.0 | 0 | 0.3 | 3 |
| lentils, boiled, 1 cup | 230 | 0.8 | 0% | 0.1 | 0.1 | 0.3 | 0 | 15.6 | 4 |
| lettuce, butter, raw, 2 leaves | 2 | 0 | 0% | 0.0 | 0.0 | 0.0 | 0 | 0.1 | 1 |
| mushrooms, ½ cup | 9 | 0.1 | 10% | 0.0 | 0.0 | 0.1 | 0 | 0.4 | 2 |
| olives, black, pitted, 2 olives | 25 | 2 | 72% | 0.0 | 1.8 | 0.0 | 0 | 0.2 | 115 |
| onions, raw, chopped, ½ cup | 30 | 0.1 | 3% | 0.0 | 0.0 | 0.0 | 0 | 1.4 | 2 |
| peas, frozen, ½ cup boiled | 62 | 0.2 | 3% | 0.0 | 0.0 | 0.1 | 0 | 4.4 | 70 |
| peas, dried split peas, ¼ cup | 110 | 0 | 0% | 0 | 0 | 0 | 0 | 11 | 25 |

| | *calories* | *total fat g* | *% of calories* | *saturated g* | *monounsatt g* | *polyunsat g* | *cholesterol mg* | *fiber g* | *sodium mg* |
|---|---|---|---|---|---|---|---|---|---|
| peppers, bell, ½ cup raw | 14 | 0.1 | 6% | 0.0 | 0.0 | 0.1 | 0 | 0.9 | 1 |
| pepper, yellow, 1 raw | 50 | 0.4 | 7% | 0.0 | 0.0 | 0.1 | 0 | 1.7 | 1 |
| potatoes, 1 raw, 4 oz | 88 | 0.1 | 1% | 0.0 | 0.0 | 0.1 | 0 | 1.8 | 7 |
| potatoes, mashed, dry, 3 tablespoons | 80 | 0.5 | 6% | 0.5 | 0.0 | 0.0 | 0 | 2.0 | 270 |
| rutabaga, boiled, ½ cup cubes | 33 | 0.2 | 5% | 0 | 0 | 0.1 | 0 | 1.5 | 17 |
| shallot, 1 tablespoon raw | 7 | 0 | 0% | 0.0 | 0.0 | 0.0 | 0 | | 1 |
| spinach, ½ cup raw, chopped | 6 | 0 | 0% | 0.0 | 0.0 | 0.0 | 0 | 0.8 | 2 |
| squash, zucchini, ½ cup raw | 9 | 0 | 0% | 0.0 | 0.0 | 0.0 | 0 | 0.8 | 3 |
| squash, yellow crookneck | 12 | 0.2 | 15% | 0.0 | 0.0 | 0.2 | 0 | 1.2 | 1 |
| squash, butternut, ½ cup baked | 41 | 0.1 | 2% | 0.0 | 0.0 | 0.1 | 0 | 4.5 | 2 |
| squash, acorn, ½ cup baked | 57 | 0.1 | 2% | 0.0 | 0.0 | 0.0 | 0 | 4.5 | 4 |
| sweet potato, 4 oz baked | 130 | 0.1 | 1% | 0.0 | 0.0 | 0.1 | 0 | 3.4 | 11 |
| tofu, raw firm, ½ cup | 183 | 11 | 54% | 1.6 | 2.4 | 6.2 | 0 | 2.9 | 18 |
| tomatoes, stewed, canned, ½ cup | 36 | 0.2 | 5% | 0.0 | 0.0 | 0.1 | 0 | 1.3 | 280 |
| tomatoes, diced, canned, ½ cup | 25 | 0 | 0% | 0.0 | 0.0 | 0.0 | 0 | 0.5 | 250 |
| tomato, 1 raw, 4 oz | 26 | 0.4 | 14% | 0.1 | 0.1 | 0.2 | 0 | 1.4 | 11 |
| tomato paste 2 tablespoons | 30 | 0 | 0% | 0.0 | 0.0 | 0.0 | 0 | 1.0 | 20 |
| tomatoes, sun-dried, 1 oz | 90 | 0 | 0% | 0.0 | 0.0 | 0.0 | 0 | 4.0 | 90 |
| **Fruit** | | | | | | | | | |
| apple, raw, medium | 81 | 0.5 | 6% | 0.1 | 0.0 | 0.2 | 0 | 3.7 | 1 |
| banana, 1 raw | 105 | 0.5 | 4% | 0.2 | 0.0 | 0.1 | 0 | 2.7 | 1 |
| blueberries, raw, 1 cup | 81 | 0.6 | 7% | 0.0 | 0.1 | 0.2 | 0 | 3.9 | 9 |
| blackberries, raw, 1 cup | 74 | 0.3 | 4% | 0.0 | 0.0 | 0.2 | 0 | 7.6 | 1 |
| cherries, raw 10 | 49 | 0.7 | 13% | 0.1 | 0.2 | 0.2 | 0 | 1.1 | 2 |
| grapes, raw, 1 cup | 58 | 0.3 | 5% | 0.1 | 0.0 | 0.1 | 0 | 0.9 | 2 |

| | *calories* | *total fat g* | *% of calories* | *saturated g* | *monounsatt g* | *polyunsat g* | *cholesterol mg* | *fiber g* | *sodium mg* |
|---|---|---|---|---|---|---|---|---|---|
| lemon juice, fresh, 1 tablespoon | 4 | 0 | 0% | 0.0 | 0.0 | 0.0 | 0 | 0.1 | 0 |
| orange juice, fresh, 8 oz | 112 | 0.5 | 4% | 0.1 | 0.1 | 0.1 | 0 | 0.1 | 2 |
| orange, raw, 1 medium | 59 | 0.4 | 6% | 0.0 | 0.1 | 0.1 | 0 | 3.1 | 1 |
| pineapple, raw, 1 cup | 76 | 0.7 | 8% | 0.0 | 0.1 | 0.2 | 0 | 1.9 | 2 |
| raspberries, raw, 1 cup | 60 | 0.7 | 10% | 0.0 | 0.1 | 0.4 | 0 | 8.4 | 0 |
| strawberries, raw, 1 cup | 45 | 0.6 | 10% | 0.0 | 0.1 | 0.3 | 0 | 3.4 | 1 |
| watermelon, raw, 1 cup | 51 | 0.7 | 11% | 0.1 | 0.2 | 0.2 | 0 | 0.8 | 3 |
| **Nuts** | | | | | | | | | |
| almonds, dry roasted, 1 oz (24 nuts) | 166 | 14.6 | 80% | 1.4 | 9.5 | 3.1 | 0 | 3.9 | 3 |
| peanuts, dry roasted, 1 oz (39 nuts) | 170 | 14.0 | 78% | 2.0 | 7.0 | 4.0 | 0 | 2.0 | 0 |
| peanut butter, 1 tablespoon | 180 | 16.3 | 82% | 3..3 | 7.8 | 4.4 | 0 | 0.7 | 214 |
| pecans, dry roasted, 1 oz (31 nuts) | 189 | 19.2 | 84% | 1.5 | 11.4 | 4.5 | 0 | 2.6 | 0 |
| **Dairy Products** | | | | | | | | | |
| butter, unsalted, 1 tablespoon | 108 | 12.2 | 100% | 7.6 | 3.5 | .5 | 33 | 0.0 | 1 |
| cottage cheese, nonfat, ½ cup | 90 | 0 | 0% | 0 | 0 | 0 | 0 | 0 | 360 |
| milk, powdered, nonfat 3 tablespoons | 80 | 0.5 | 6% | 0.4 | 0.1 | 0.0 | 1 | 0.0 | 125 |
| milk, nonfat, 8 oz | 86 | 0.4 | 4% | 0.3 | 0.1 | 0.0 | 4 | 0.0 | 125 |
| milk, 2%, 8 oz | 121 | 4.7 | 35% | 2.9 | 1.4 | 0.2 | 18 | 0.0 | 122 |
| milk, 3.7% (whole), 8 oz | 157 | 8.9 | 51% | 5.6 | 2.6 | 0.3 | 35 | 0.0 | 119 |
| yogurt, nonfat, 1 cup | 110 | 0 | 0% | 0.0 | 0.0 | 0.0 | 0 | 0.0 | 160 |
| yogurt, frozen, nonfat, 1 cup | 180 | 0 | 0% | 0.0 | 0.0 | 0.0 | 0 | 0.0 | 100 |

| | *calories* | *total fat g* | *% of calories* | *saturated g* | *monounsatt g* | *polyunsat g* | *cholesterol mg* | *fiber g* | *sodium mg* |
|---|---|---|---|---|---|---|---|---|---|
| **Fish** | | | | | | | | | |
| halibut, 4 oz | 120 | 1.9 | 14% | 0.5 | 0.8 | 0.8 | 34 | 0.0 | 60 |
| oysters, Pacific, raw, 3 oz | 69 | 2 | 26% | 0.4 | 0.3 | 0.8 | 43 | 0.0 | 90 |
| sablefish, 4 oz | 210 | 20 | 86% | 5.0 | 10.0 | 3.0 | 50 | 0.0 | 60 |
| salmon, 4 oz | 160 | 5.4 | 30% | 1.0 | 2.2 | 2.6 | 50 | 0.0 | 60 |
| sea bass, 4 oz | 105 | 1.7 | 15% | 0.5 | 0.5 | 0.8 | 44 | 0.0 | 72 |
| scallops, 4 oz | 60 | 0.7 | 11% | 0.1 | 0.1 | 0.0 | 34 | 0.0 | 50 |
| shrimp, 4 oz | 122 | 2 | 15% | 0.4 | 0.3 | 0.8 | 25 | 0.0 | 126 |
| calamari, 4 oz | 100 | 1.2 | 11% | 0.4 | 0.2 | 0.4 | 240 | 0.0 | 46 |
| swordfish, 4 oz | 128 | 4 | 28% | 1.1 | 1.7 | 1.1 | 40 | 0.0 | 90 |
| tuna, raw, 4 oz | 112 | 1.1 | 9% | 0.2 | 0.1 | 0.2 | 47 | 0.0 | 31 |
| tuna canned in water, 4 oz | 140 | 1.5 | 10% | 0.0 | 0.9 | 0.6 | 40 | 0.0 | 400 |
| **Poultry** | | | | | | | | | |
| chicken breast, 4 oz | 130 | 3.1 | 21% | 0.9 | 1.1 | 0.7 | 73 | 0.0 | 64 |
| chicken broth, 1 cup | 10 | 0 | 0% | 0.0 | 0.0 | 0.0 | 0 | 0.0 | 570 |
| egg substitute, ¼ cup | 35 | 0 | 0% | 0.0 | 0.0 | 0.0 | 0 | 0.0 | 160 |
| turkey breast, nonfat, 4 oz | 104 | 0.4 | 3% | 0.2 | 0.2 | 0.1 | 23 | 0.0 | 76 |
| **Oil and Wine** | | | | | | | | | |
| canola oil, 1 tablespoon | 124 | 14 | 102% | 1.0 | 8.2 | 4.1 | 0 | 0.0 | 0 |
| olive oil, 1 tablespoon | 124 | 14 | 102% | 1.9 | 10.3 | 1.2 | 0 | 0.0 | 0 |
| sesame oil, 1 tablespoon | 124 | 14 | 102% | 2.0 | 5.6 | 5.8 | 0 | 0.0 | 0 |
| wine, 12%, 4 oz | 82 | 0 | 0% | 0.0 | 0.0 | 0.0 | 0 | 0.0 | 6 |
| **Other** | | | | | | | | | |
| bagel, 3 oz | 195 | 1.1 | 5% | 0.2 | 0.1 | 0.5 | 0 | 1.6 | 379 |
| beer, Budweiser, 12 oz | 147 | 0 | 0% | 0.0 | 0.0 | 0.0 | 0 | 0.0 | 12 |
| Big Mac, McDonald's | 560 | 32.4 | 52% | 10.1 | 20.9 | 1.5 | 103 | 2.0 | 950 |
| cheeseburger, dbl bacon Burger King | 640 | 39 | 55% | 18.0 | | | 145 | 2.0 | 1240 |

| | *calories* | *total fat g* | *% of calories* | *saturated g* | *monounsatt g* | *polyunsat g* | *cholesterol mg* | *fiber g* | *sodium mg* |
|---|---|---|---|---|---|---|---|---|---|
| chocolate chips, Hershey 1 tablespoon | 80 | 4.3 | 48% | 2.7 | 0.0 | 0.0 | 1 | 0.0 | 2 |
| doughnut, glazed | 192 | 10.3 | 48% | 2.4 | 5.4 | 1.2 | 14 | 0.7 | 181 |
| English muffin, Thomas, 2 oz | 138 | 1 | 7% | 0.1 | 0.2 | 0.5 | 0 | 1.8 | 193 |
| French fries, McDonald's, 4.3 oz | 400 | 21.6 | 49% | 9.1 | 11.6 | 0.9 | 16 | 3.0 | 200 |
| ice cream Haagen-Dazs, 1 cup | 286 | 14.6 | 46% | 9.0 | 4.2 | 0.6 | 44 | 0.0 | 100 |
| ketchup, 1 tablespoon | 15 | 0 | 0% | 0.0 | 0.0 | 0.0 | 0 | 0.0 | 190 |
| Pepsi, 12 oz | 150 | 0 | 0% | 0.0 | 0.0 | 0.0 | 0 | 0.0 | 4 |
| pizza, 1/8 of 12" w cheese, meat | 140 | 7 | 45% | 2.2 | 3.1 | 1.2 | 14 | 2.0 | 267 |
| steak, tenderloin, 10 oz | 900 | 62 | 62% | 24.0 | 25.0 | 2.4 | 250 | 0.0 | 180 |
| Whopper, double, Burger King | 870 | 56 | 58% | 19.0 | | | 170 | 3.0 | 940 |

# *Authors*

Blair Beebe, MD, MLA, FACP, has been associate executive director of the Permanente Medical Group, Kaiser Permanente, and physician-in-chief of Santa Teresa Hospital, San Jose, California. He is board certified in internal medicine, a fellow of the American College of Physicians, and a former clinical faculty member in the Department of Endocrinology and Metabolism at Stanford University. He recently received a master of liberal arts degree from Stanford. He has also been a member of the Medial Advisory Committee of the Technology Evaluation Center sponsored by the Blue Cross/Blue Shield Association in Chicago, and a senior clinical consultant to Computer Sciences Corporation.

Sue Beebe, MA, has a master's degree in microbiology and an interest in nutrition on a cellular basis that stems from studying microorganisms. In the past, she has taught nursing students at two local community colleges and at San Jose State University. She has attended three cooking schools in France: Lenôtre and Marguerite's in Paris, and l'École des Trois Ponts in Roanne. A longtime fan of Julia Child and Ina Garten, she has incorporated the principles outlined by the Nutritional Guidelines for Americans into their culinary concepts.

# *References*

Antman, E. M. and E. Braumwald. 2001. "Acute Myocardial Infarction." *Harrison's Principles of Internal Medicine.* 15th Edition. Chapter 243. http://www.harrisononline.com/.

Appel, L. J., et al. 1997. "A Clinical Trial of the Effects of Dietary Patterns on Blood Pressure." *New England Journal of Medicine.* Vol: 336 (16), 1117–1124.

Baker, J. L., et al. 2007. "Childhood Body-Mass Index and the Risk of Coronary Heart Disease in Adulthood." *New England Journal of Medicine.* Vol: 357 (23), 2329–2327.

Barter, P., et al. 2007. "HDL Cholesterol, Very Low Levels of LDL Cholesterol, and Cardiovascular Events." *New England Journal of Medicine.* Vol: 357 (13), 1301.

Bartolucci, A. A., and G. Howard. 2006. "Meta-analysis of data from the six primary prevention trials of cardiovascular events using aspirin." *American Journal of Cardiology.* Vol: 98 (6), 746–750.

Bibbins-Domingo, K., et al., 2007. "Adolescent Overweight and Future Adult Coronary Heart Disease." *New England Journal of Medicine.* Vol: 357 (23), 2371–2379.

Breslow, J. L. 2006. "N-3 Fatty Acids and Cardiovascular Disease." *American Journal of Clinical Nutrition.* Vol: 83 (6 Suppl), 1477S–1482S.

Brunzell, J. D., 2007. "Hypertriglyceridemia." *New England Journal of Medicine.* Vol: 357 (10), 1009–1017.

"Bulletin of the World Health Organization. 2007. Vol: 85 (6), 474–481.

Christakis, N. A., and J. H. Fowler. 2007. "The Spread of Obesity in a Large Social Network over 32 Years." *New England Journal of Medicine.* Vol: 357 (4), 370.

Cucciolla V., et al. 2007. "Resveratrol: from Basic Science to the Clinic." *Cell Cycle.* Vol: 6 (20), 2495–2510.

Dansinger, M. L., et al. 2005. "Comparison of the Atkins, Ornish, Weight Watchers, and Zone Diets for Weight Loss and Heart Disease Risk Reduction." *Journal of the American Medical Association.* Vol: 293, 43–53.

Demetrius, L. 2006. "Aging in Mouse and Human Systems: A Comparative Study." *Annals of the New York Academy of Science.* Vol: 1067, 66–82.

De Wals, P., et al. 2007. "Reduction in Neural-Tube Defects after Folic Acid Fortification in Canada." *New England Journal of Medicine.* Vol: 357 (2), 135.

Domanski, M. J. 2007. "Primary Prevention of Coronary Artery Disease." *New England Journal of Medicine.* Vol: 357 (15), 1543.

Duffy, S. W., et al. 2002. "The Impact of Organized Mammography Service Screening on Breast Carcinoma Mortality in Seven Swedish Counties." *Cancer.* Vol: 95 (3), 458–459.

Espin, J. C., et al. 2007. "Nutraceuticals: Facts and Fiction." *Phytochemistry.* Vol: 68 (22-24), 2986–3008.

Folsom, A. R. 2007. "Degree of Concordance with DASH Diet Guidelines and Incidence of Hypertension and Fatal Cardiovascular Disease." *American Journal of Hypertension.* Vol: 20 (3), 223.

Ford, I., et al. 2007. "Long-Term Follow-up of the West of Scotland Coronary Prevention Study." *New England Journal of Medicine.* Vol: 357 (15), 1477.

Ford, S., et al. 2007. "Explaining the Decrease in U.S. Deaths from Coronary Disease, 1980–2000." *New England Journal of Medicine.* Vol: 356 (23), 2388.

Ginsberg, H. N. and I. J. Goldberg. *Harrison's Principles of Internal Medicine.* Version 1.0. McGraw-Hill, Table 344–2. 2001. CD-ROM.

Grimley, M. M., et al., 2003. "Folic Acid with or without Vitamin B12 for Cognition and Dementia." *Cochrane Database System Review.* Vol: 4, CD004514.

Hansen, A.S., et al. 2005. "Effect of Red Wine and Red Grape Extract on Blood Lipids, Haemostatic Factors, and Other Risk Factors for Cardiovascular Disease." European Journal of Clinical Nutrition. Vol: 59 (3), 449–55.

Hooper, L., R. L. Thompson, R. A. Harrison, R.A., et al. 2006. "Risks and Benefits of Omega-3 fats for Mortality, Cardiovascular Disease, and Cancer: Systematic Review." *British Medical Journal.* Vol: 332, 752–760.

Hu, F. B. 2003. "The Mediterranean Diet and Mortality—Olive Oil and Beyond." *New England Journal of Medicine.* Vol: 348 (26), 2595–2596.

Kelly, S. A. 2007. "Whole grain Cereals for Coronary Heart Disease." *Cochrane Database System Review.* CD005051.

Kereiakes, D. J., et al. 2007. "The Truth and Consequences of the COURAGE trial." *Journal of the American College of Cardiology.* Vol: 50 (16), 1598–1603.

Kinsella, K. G. 2005. "Future Longevity-Demographic Concerns and Consequences." *Journal of the American Geriatrics Society.* Vol: 53 (9 Suppl), S299–S303.

Koek, H. L., et. al. 2007. "Incidence of First Acute Myocardial Infarction in the Netherlands." *Netherlands Journal of Medicine.* Vol: 65 (11), 434–441.

Lee, I. M., et al., 2005. "Vitamin E in the Primary Prevention of Cardiovascular Disease and Cancer: the Women's Health Study: a Randomized Controlled Trial." *Journal of the American Medical Association.* Vol: 294 (1), 56–65.

Lemaitre, R. N., et al. 2003. "N-3 Polyunsaturated Fatty Acids, Fatal Ischemic Heart disease, and Nonfatal Myocardial Infarction in Older Adults : the Cardiovascular Health Study." *American Journal of Clinical Nutrition.* Vol: 77 (2), 319–325.

Louria, D. B. 2005. "Extraordinary Longevity: Individual and Societal Issues." *Journal of the American Geriatrics Society.* Vol: 53 (9 Suppl), S317–S319.

Ludwig, D. S. 2007. "Childhood Obesity—The Shape of Things to Come." *New England Journal of Medicine.* Vol: 357 (23), 2325–2327.

Mathers, C. D., et al. June 2000. "Estimates of DALE for 191 Countries, Methods and Results." World Health Organization. p. 51. http://www.who.int/healthinfo/paper16pdf.

Mozaffarian, D., et al. 2005. "Interplay Between Different Polyunsaturated Fatty Acids and Risk of Coronary Heart Disease in Men." *Circulation.* Vol: 111 (2), 157–164.

Mozaffarian, D., et al. 2006. "Trans Fatty Acids and Cardiovascular Disease." *The New England Journal of Medicine.* Vol: 354 (15), 1601–1613.

National Heart, Lung, and Blood Institute. American Heart Association. National Institutes of Health. National Cholesterol Education Program. 2007. http://www.nhlbi.nih.gov/chd/.

National Vital Statistics Reports. 2006. Vol: 54 (16) and (14) Table 11.

Noda, H., et al. 2008. "Smoking Status, Sports Participation and Mortality from Coronary Heart Disease." *Heart.* Vol: 94 (4), 471–475).

Ogden, C. L., et al. 2006. "Prevalence of Overweight and Obesity in the United States, 1999–2004." *Journal of the American Medical Association.* Vol: 295 (13), 1549–1555.

Oh, R. 2008. "Hypertriglyceridemia." *The New England Journal of Medicine.* Vol: 358 (3), 310.

Olshansky, S. J., et al. 1990. "In Search of Methuselah: Estimating the Upper Limits to Human Longevity." *Science.* Vol: 250 (4981), 634–640.

Olshansky, S. J., et al. 2005. "A Potential Decline in Life Expectancy in the United States in the 21st Century." *New England Journal of Medicine.* Vol: 352 (11), 1138–1145.

Pennington, J. A. 1998. *Bowes & Church's Food Values of Portions Commonly Used.* Philadelphia: Lippincott, 110-118.

Ridker, P. M. 2005. "A Randomized Trial of Low-dose Aspirin in the Primary Prevention of Cardiovascular Disease in Women." *New England Journal of Medicine.* Vol: 352 (13), 1293–1304.

Ryan-Harshman, M. 2007. "Diet and Colorectal Cancer: Review of the Evidence." *Canadian Family Physician.* Vol: 53 (11), 1913–1920.

Saiko, P., et al. 2007. "Resveratrol and its Analogs: Defense Against Cancer Coronary Disease and Neurodegenerative Maladies or Just a Fad?" *Mutation Research.* Vol: 658 (1–2), 68–94)

Seal, C. J. 2006. "Whole Grains and CVD risk." *Proceedings of the Nutrition Society.* Vol: 65 (1), 24–34.

Sesso, H. D., R. S. Paffenbarger, Jr, and I. M. Lee. 2000. "Physical Activity and Coronary Heart Disease in Men: The Harvard Alumni Study." *Circulation.* Vol: 102 (9).

Shai, Iris. 2008. "Weight Loss with a Low-Carbohydrate, Mediterranean, or Low-Fat Diet." New England Journal of Medicine. Vol: 359 (3), 229–41.

Sizer, F. S., and E. N. Whitney. 1994. *Hamilton and Whitney's Nutrition, Concepts and Controversies.* St. Paul: West. 106.

Stryer, Lubert. 1981. *Biochemistry.* 2nd Ed. New York: Freeman. 226–227.

Sytkowski, P. A., W. B. Kannel, R. B. D'Agostino. 1990. "Changes in Risk Factors and the Decline in Mortality from Cardiovascular Disease. The Framingham Heart Study." *New England Journal of Medicine.* Vol: 322 (23), 1635–41.

Tanasescu, M., et al. 2003. "Exercise Type and Intensity in Relation to Coronary Heart Disease in Men. *Journal of the American Medical Association.* Vol: 288 (16), 1994–2000.

Thadani, U. 2004. "Current Medical Management of Chronic Stable Angina." *Journal of Cardiovascular Pharmacologic Therapy.* Vol: 9, (1 Suppl), S11–29.

Truswell, A. S. 2002. "Cereal Grains and Coronary Heart Disease." *European Journal of Clinical Nutrition.* Vol: 56 (1), 1–14.

Tu, Jack V., et al. 1997. "Use of Cardiac Procedures and Outcomes in Elderly Patients with Myocardial Infarction in the United States and

Canada." *New England Journal of Medicine.* Vol: 336 (21), 1500 –1505.

United States Department of Agriculture and the Department of Health and Human Services. 2005. "Dietary Guidelines Advisory Committee Report." http://www.health.gov/dietary guidelines/dga2005/report/default.htm.

U. S. Preventive Services Task Force. 2007. "Screening for Carotid Artery Stenosis: USPSTF Recommendation Statement." *Annals of Internal Medicine,* Vol: 147 (12), 854–859.

Unützer, J. 2007. "Late-Life Depression." *New England Journal of Medicine.* Vol: 357 (22), 269–276.

van der Worp, H. P. and J. van Gijn. 2007. "Acute Ischemic Stroke." *New England Journal of Medicine.* Vol: 357 (6), 572–578.

Vogel, R.A. 2002. "Alcohol, Heart Disease, and Mortality: A Review." Review Cardiovascular Medicine. Vol: 3 (1), 7–13.

Walsh, P. C., T. L. DeWeese, M. A. Eisenberger. 2007. "Localized Prostate Cancer." *New England Journal of Medicine.* Vol: 357 (26), 2696–2705.

Weintraub, W.S., et al. 2008. "Effect of PCI on Quality of Life in Patients with Stable Coronary Disease." New England Journal of Medicine. Vol: 359 (7), 677–87.

Willcox, B. J., et al., 2007. "Caloric Restriction, the Traditional Okinawan Diet, and Healthy Aging: The Diet of the World's Longest-Lived People and Its Potential Impact on Morbidity and Life Span." *Annals of the New York Academy of Science.* Vol: 1114, 434–455.

Willet, W. C. 1995. "Mediterranean Diet Pyramid: A Cultural Model for Healthy Eating. *American Journal of Clinical Nutrition.* Vol: 61, (Suppl), 1402S–1406S.

Willet, W. C. 2007. "The Role of Dietary n-6 Fatty Acids in the Prevention of Cardiovascular Disease." *Journal of Cardiovascular Medicine* (Hagerstown). Vol: 8, (1 Suppl), S42–45.

Williamson, J. D., and L. P. Fried. 1996. "Characterization of Older Adults who Attribute Functional Decrements to Old Age." *Journal of the American Geriatrics Society.* Vol: 44 (12), 1429–1434.

Wilmoth, J. R. 2000. "Demography of Longevity: Past, Present, and Future Trends." *Experimental Gerontology.* Vol: 35 (9–10), 1111–1129.

World Health Organization. 2008, "Data and Statistics." http://www.who.int/research/en/.

Wu, J. M., et al. 2001. "Mechanism of Cardioprotection by Resveratrol, a Phenolic Antioxidant Present in Red Wine." *International Journal of Molecular Medicine.* Vol: 8 (1), 3–17.

Yusuf, S., et al. 2000. "Vitamin E Supplementation and Cardiovascular Events in High-risk Patients. The Heart Outcomes Prevention Evaluation Study Investigators." *New England Journal of Medicine.* Vol: 342 (3), 154–160.

# *Index*

## C



## D



## E

## F



## G



## H



## I

**K**



**L**



**M**



**N**



**O**

**P**

## R



## S

**T**



**U**



**V**

**W**



**Y**



**Z**